The Pants

"Get up! It's finally here!"

It was a crisp Chicago morning, and my blood was pumping. I jumped out of bed. "It's today! It's here!"

I nudged my groggy and not-so-enthused husband. "Uppy, uppy, little puppy."

He moaned and mumbled something about five more minutes. I was used to his lack of springiness in the morning, so I'd worked in three "five more minutes" as a buffer. He rolled over and started snoring instantly.

"Let's check the bags one more time," I said, only to receive a sleepy "but we've checked the bags ten times and it's just a weekend trip." I would not be deterred.

I plopped the oversized black suitcase onto our oversized comforter. "Friday pants and shirt…check. Saturday-day shirt and comfy jeans…kinda check." I was going to wear my favorite comfy jeans on the plane. You know those jeans—they fit like a glove, they stretch and move with you like a second skin, and they make you feel great. You own the world in those jeans. You're invincible in those jeans.

"Saturday-night shirt and dressy, not as comfy jeans." These were the jeans that made my ass look perky. A must if we hit the town. I mean, it was a new city—I had to look the part.

"Comfy sweats and T-shirt for the flight back…check. Way too many pairs of panties…check." Um, ten pairs of panties for a three-day trip, just in case? Just in case what? I'd always done this. Was it because I'd worked at Victoria's Secret in college? What could possibly happen that I'd need seven extra pairs of panties?

Focus.

"Makeup…check. Contacts, an extra pair, solution, case, glasses…check. Comfy shoes…check. Not so comfy (will kill my feet by the end of the night, in fact) but really cute shoes…check. Toothbrush and toothpaste…check." *Do I need to lug floss around on the trip? Will it be the end of the world if I skipped flossing for a weekend?* No check for floss.

"Hair products to tame my wild curls…check." I'd been blessed with hair that worked in a scrunch-and-go style. I love it now but as a schoolgirl I hated it. I wanted straight blonde hair, like Stacy. You know this hair and this girl. She always looked flawless.

"Okay, I think that's it!"

I flopped myself over the suitcase's top and pushed, zipped, pushed, zipped, pushed, and zipped as the zipper held on for dear life. Finally, I claimed victory.

T-minus four hours until departure.

I'm one of those crazy people who needs to be at the airport at least two hours early. In my defense, have you ever tried to get through Chicago's O'Hare airport in less than two hours? It's crazy busy, and if you don't keep moving, you'll get trampled. Weirdly, it's still one of my favorite airports.

In the shower, I felt nervousness settle in. This wasn't just any old weekend trip. In six short weeks, my husband and I would be moving to Raleigh, North Carolina. I'd received a big promotion at the boutique recruiting agency I worked for and would now be running the Raleigh branch. And this weekend was our only chance to find a place to rent. On top of all that crazy, I was turning thirty over the weekend.

Would I fit in in the South? I wondered. Would people judge me because I didn't like shrimp and grits and sweet tea? Would they find my directness offensive? Or would they love me? Would these be my people—the people I'd been trying to find a place with my whole life? I'd always had a small group of wonderful friends but had never felt like I was part of a group. I'd always felt like an outsider looking in. I envied people who seemed to fit in perfectly anywhere, chameleon-like.

I couldn't deny I was nervous to move almost a thousand miles away from home. The furthest I'd ventured was in college, when I lived three hours away. And even then, I went home most weekends—I've always been ridiculously close to my mom, who raised me as a single mother. She's my sounding board, my best friend, and my biggest supporter, even when I'm doing something stupid and she doesn't agree with it (like when I dated that idiot back in college—she never even pulled out the big fat "I told you so!").

This is it, I told myself as I rinsed the suds from my hair. *You just need to get ready and go.*

I grabbed my soft, baggy black T-shirt. There was once a time in my life when I should have owned stock in Old Navy and the Gap. I owned every soft cotton shirt they made. They were the go-to in my daily wardrobe.

My favorite jeans were ready on the bench at the foot of the bed, folded neatly in the three-crease style that I'd perfected during my college internship at the Gap. If I'd learned anything in my time there, it was how to fold the crap out of everything.

I missed wearing my favorite jeans; in my job, the dress code was business casual with an emphasis on *business*. I spent most weekdays in tight, uncomfortable dress pants and most weekends unwinding in yoga pants, so it had been a while since my trusty pair of jeans had been out in the world.

Getting to this point in my career had been an interesting road, to say the least. After college, at twenty-three years old, I'd struggled to find my footing in a career. My degree in fashion merchandising seemed useless, and I wasn't ready to leave the nest for anything more than a thirty-minute drive. And so, the onslaught of shitty jobs began.

First, I sold online college programs for a college that turned out to not be accredited. Then I worked for a title company preparing reports about houses that weren't in flood zones, and I worked for a time typing up mold remediation reports.

A year later, I said *screw this* and started my own business making bath-bomb cupcakes (more about that later). Four and a half years and one recession later, I closed the business that I loved and had grown to eight employees and took the job that would change my life in so many ways—the job that would become a career that, frankly, I fucking rock at. The job that would take me to North Carolina.

They say every decision we make alters the course of our lives. Applying for an entry-level, mostly commission-based job that quite honestly sounded like a scam was one of the biggest decisions I ever made. I called my bestie and told her I was going to try it until I found a "real" job. Eleven years later, I'd hired over five hundred people and was working globally as a talent acquisition manager (aka recruiter).

And for this career, I had to dress the part. So, I was excited about the prospect of a weekend with my trusty jeans.

I grabbed the first leg and put my foot through. I grabbed the other leg and put my other foot through. Then I slid the jeans over my knees and past my upper thighs. The farther up I went, the tighter they got—tighter than I remembered. I did a wiggly squat to hoist them up.

No such luck. Time to bring in the reinforcements. I hooked my thumbs through the beltloops and began to pull.

Pull, wiggle, pull, jump, wiggle, squat. Wiggle, wiggle, pull. *Did someone dry my favorite comfy pants? On high heat? My fat pants?* Squat, pull, pull. *OMG, am I starting to breathe heavily? Is that sweat pouring down my face or are those tears? Do NOT cry, do NOT cry.*

There are two types of criers in the world: the Miss-America-receiving-her-crown crier and the ugly crier. I am the latter. When I cry, which isn't often, my eyes get red and puffy, my whole face turns a shade of red similar to a fire truck, and snot streams out of my nose like a faucet (and not a leaky, dripping faucet but a busted-pipe-water-everywhere faucet). And the best part: I look this way for hours.

Choking back the tears, I focused on happy thoughts, and after several more minutes of lying on the floor and sucking in my stomach, I secured the button. My jeans were on. Finally.

I resolved not to let this minor setback ruin my weekend.

At the airport, we headed up to a kiosk to print our tickets—this was before the era of smartphones, so we were rocking travel old-school style. As I looked around, I wondered if the apocalypse had happened without our knowledge. Where were all the people? The lines, the chaos, the confusion? I was waiting for tumbleweeds to blow through the terminal, like in an old Clint Eastwood Western. Maybe this was a sign from the travel gods: the near meltdown over my pants was a blip, and the trip would be nothing but smooth sailing from here on out.

After breezing through security, my husband and I plotted our airport-breakfast extravaganza. *Extravaganza* is really the only word that accurately described the time we spent eating. We both struggled with our weight, and we leaned on each other, silently confirming to each other that our behavior was appropriate. Food was a source of happiness. And, well, involved a lot of shitty choices.

That morning, I wolfed down two breakfast burritos and a Frappuccino, the nectar of the gods. Afterward, feeling overstuffed and tired, I looked forward to taking an hour-and-a-half-long catnap on the plane.

Finally on board, I "excuse me, sorry, excuse me, sorry" shuffled through the narrow aisle. When had planes gotten so small? I was pretty sure I'd whacked two people in the head with my carry-on bag along the way, but that's all part of the travel fun, right?

The plane was one of those big but not really big ones that has two seats on the left side and three on the right side. I was grateful we were on the two-seater side and wouldn't have to share the space with a stranger. We all have nightmare plane stories—like sitting next to a person who takes off their shoes so their feet can "breathe," or an over-talker, or a snorer, or sitting in front of a kid who kicks your seat. Having retrieved my iPod Nano and book and magazine and neck pillow and gum and water from my carry-on, I settled into my seat. All set. Just needed to buckle in.

I grabbed the left side of the belt and then the right. They didn't reach each other. *Hmmm.* I lengthened the right side. They still didn't reach. Maybe my husband and I had our belts mixed up and he was sitting on mine?

"Get up, you're sitting on my belt!"

He frowned at me with annoyance. "No I'm not. I'm already belted in."

"You can't be because mine isn't working, so the pieces must be mixed up." I took a closer look at his seat belt. Sure enough, he was belted in correctly. How could an airline be operating with faulty seat belts?

I flagged down the flight attendant who looked like a young Sharon Stone.

"May I help you?" she asked, in a sweet Southern accent.

"Yes, my seat belt is broken. Do I need to move seats?"

She examined the seat belt as I showed her how the pieces just wouldn't connect. Then she looked at me. Looked at the seat belt again.

"I'll be right back," she said in a low voice. "Just hang tight." She walked away, and I watched her whisper with an older flight attendant. At one point, they looked at me with sad, almost pitiful expressions.

Moments later, the young flight attendant returned. "Honey, there's nothing wrong with the belt—you just need a little extra help." She passed something to me. "Here's a seat-belt extender."

Her words came out in slow motion. It was like in the movies when everything comes to a screeching halt. I could hear what she was saying, but I didn't understand what it meant. A seat-belt extender? Was this some type of tiny plane? Was everyone else having this issue? Why wasn't anyone else complaining about their super-small seat belt?

I clicked it into place, looked out of the window, and burst into the ugliest tears you've ever seen.

My husband had no idea what to do. Remember, I'm not a crier. "Are you okay?"

I couldn't respond; I had no words. I continued facing the window and used the sleeve of my favorite black sweater to wipe away the tears and snot streaming down my face. This was supposed to have been the start of the best weekend and there I was, ugly-crying in the pants that I'd barely been able to get on. And along for the ride was my new travel companion—the seat-belt extender.

It was the lowest point of my life.

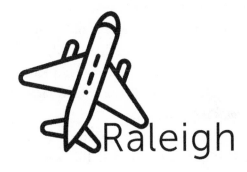

Raleigh

As we hit the tarmac, I flew forward. A combination of the morning's overwhelming emotions and the plane's humming had put me to sleep, mouth wide open. Dazed and confused, I wiped the drool dripping down the side of my ugly-cry face.

It had all been a nightmare, right?

I looked down and there it was in neon flashing lights: the extender, mocking me. *Fatty fat fat fat!*

How had I gotten to this point? I'd known I was a little overweight, but overweight enough to need a seat-belt extender? I wondered if I had some sort of reverse positive body image, where I looked in the mirror and saw a thinner version of myself. There had been times when I looked in the mirror and thought, *Dang, I look good*, only to later see a picture of myself taken on the same day and not even recognize myself.

Just a few weeks earlier, I'd been at a birthday party with friends and felt great. I'd rocked my favorite jeans (which apparently still fit a month and half before, kinda), my classic black T-shirt, and TOMS. When I saw pictures of the party on Facebook, I couldn't believe it was me. It seemed as if there were a fat filter on the picture.

In the photo, I wasn't wearing my favorite bracelet, the one from Tiffany & Co., which I got on my twenty-first birthday. It was silver with a little heart, like the one Reese Witherspoon wore in *Legally Blonde*. I wasn't wearing it because it didn't fit my wrist anymore. Instead, it was tucked away in a drawer. My thighs were so large they forced my feet outward and my skin looked dull, washed out. I wrote the picture off—*it's the camera angle, the way I'm leaning in, the person's shitty camera.*

I came up with a lot of reasons why that picture was so bad and denied the obvious. This was how I looked. This was who I had become.

If you're starting to think "I don't believe you can be big and beautiful or thin and ugly (both inside and out)," you're wrong. I don't think thin equals beautiful—or even healthy. I could finish a 5k race, slowly, and knew thin girls who couldn't get farther than half a mile.

Most of us have an ideal regarding who we want to be and how we want to look and feel. I've never had notions of being a size zero. Hell, I didn't have notions of being a size six. My goal at the time was simple: to shop in the same stores as my friends.

My bestie is quite the shopper, and it had always been our thing to do together. But in college I'd get so envious sitting on the bench outside the changerooms in Banana Republic or LOFT and watching her feet under the door. In her white socks, she'd turn from side to side and twirl, determining if she'd found the perfect outfit. Do you know what it's like to go to the mall and be able to shop in only one, maybe two stores that carry clothes in your size and don't make you look like you're wearing a trash bag?

Somewhere, designers decided, "She's plus-size, so she can't be sexy or sophisticated. Just make her a sack and she'll be happy it fits." It sucks. I felt shitty every time I needed a new outfit for a party or work.

My desired image largely revolved around weight but also my

health. I was slowly coming to the conclusion that I couldn't keep bingeing the way I had been without repercussions. Diabetes and heart disease would have my name written all over them if I didn't get it together.

The truth was, I depended on food. I ate to celebrate everything: promotions, big commissions, birthdays. Hell, it got to the point I was celebrating regular moments just as an excuse to overeat. But underneath, there was so much unhappiness. I ate to fill voids and satisfy emotions. I ate because I didn't think I deserved to be loved. Food became my lover, and it never let me down. It made me happy and was always there for me. Unlike the person I was in a relationship with.

A voice from the overhead speakers cut through my thoughts. "Welcome to Raleigh, the City of Oaks. The temperature is eighty-five degrees on this gorgeous October morning."

Did he just say eighty-five degrees in October? Where had we just landed, on the sun? What the hell were the summers here like if it was this warm in October? Did they even wear sweaters here? Would I have to start wearing shorts?

Did I just make a big mistake?

As the crowded plane started to empty, I stood up too quickly and fell back down into my seat. I was lightheaded—probably from all the crying. *Could I have cried out all my calories? Is that why I'm sad and hungry?*

After navigating through a much smaller and brighter airport than O'Hare, my husband and I made our way to the rental car. A weekend of house-hunting lay before us, and in North Carolina's crazy-fast market, it wouldn't be easy.

We added the first address to the GPS we'd rented for an extra ten dollars a day (again, before the days of smartphones). It was in a city called Knightdale, right outside of Raleigh. The populations in smaller towns like this one had been growing for the last few years, as it was becoming expensive and crowded within the city limits.

As we exited the airport, sunlight drenched us, almost to the point of blinding. Now I was convinced we'd landed on the sun. Trees towered over the four-lane highway, and they were just starting to change color—there were bright reds and burnt yellows. The scene was a stark contrast to the concrete jungle and smog of Chicago. I'd never realized how gray Chicago was until I saw the blue skies of North Carolina.

I tried to put the morning shenanigans behind me. I mean, there was nothing I could do at that moment to help the situation. As the realtor bounced us from apartment to house to townhouse, I took in everything around me: Was the place close to a mall? Did the area look clean and safe? How close were the nearest Targets and Starbucks?

We looked, critiqued, judged. And we learned you can get pretty good bang for your buck in Raleigh compared to Chicago and other big cities. So, we hoped to upgrade. We wanted something with a man cave for him, a craft room for me, a guest room for visitors, outdoor space for the dogs to play, and a perfect spot to entertain. I imagined throwing parties for our new friends and neighbors and hosting friends and family from back home.

"Ummm what the hell is that?"

We were in a fancy house, and I'd been daydreaming about hosting dinner parties and placing mini quiches on my perfect white serving pieces set up neatly on the granite island.

"Is that…a cockroach?"

The realtor explained that it was a palmetto bug and that they were quite common here. "Palmetto bug" is just Southern for giant flying fucking cockroach.

I screamed and jumped, nearly knocking down both my husband and the realtor in an ungraceful moment of sheer panic.

I'm not a bug person.

Once when I was in high school, I got into the shower without my glasses and thought there was a piece of brown hair near the drain. When I picked it up, I discovered it was a millipede—like, the thing with a hundred thousand legs that runs at lightning speed. I went screaming out of the shower buck naked. At least only my mom was home!

Fifteen places later, we found it—our new home. It wasn't the one with the cockroach but the first place we'd looked at. Isn't that always how it goes? It was in a cul-de-sac in a quiet subdivision where everyone had perfectly manicured lawns, where white lilies and rose bushes bloomed, and where kids rode their bikes. Had we just rented a house in the fifties?

It was the perfect shade of French blue and had gray shutters and a porch with white railings. I imagined creating a little nook in the front, where I'd have my morning coffee and read the paper. I didn't currently drink coffee or read the paper at home in the morning, but I was going to be a new and different me—dare I say a better me—in North Carolina. The inside of the house was twice as big as our townhouse in Chicago, and the tree-lined backyard seemed to go on forever. It also had the perfect open floor plan for all the entertaining we'd be doing.

We signed and officially became North Carolinians!

With all the stress of finding the right place out of the way, we ventured out to see the sights in Raleigh. The city is a beautiful place where good-old-fashioned Southern hospitality still exists. A place where people say "sir" and "ma'am" and strangers talk to you in the grocery store. But don't let this fool you. I quickly learned that "bless your heart" isn't an expression of affection but a good-old

Southern bitch slap! I guess that's where the saying "don't mess with the South" came from. Or is that "don't mess with Texas"? Either way, watch it.

The skylines of downtown Raleigh pale in comparison to the gorgeous ones of Chicago and New York. At the time, the tallest buildings couldn't have been higher than twenty, maybe twenty-five stories, and there were only a few of those. But Raleigh has a charm and personality of its own. Most of the buildings are red brick, or had been at one point, and had undergone renovation to welcome the next generation of city-goers.

As we walked through the streets trying to determine where to grab a bite, while also trying to remember what street we parked the car on and also take in all the sights and not look like tourists, I really started to look at the people. And all the emotions I'd felt earlier in the day started to creep back up.

I felt a lump in my throat. *OMG, look at these women.* They were gorgeous—slim, toned, tanned, wearing shorts that were just a little too short but still appropriate, and sporting pearly white teeth and beach-tousled hair.

Imagine a place where Reese Witherspoon, Sandra Bullock, and Scarlett Johansson are out on a Saturday evening with [insert your dream man here], eating dinner and having cocktails, laughing and being effortlessly beautiful. I mean, come on!

To make matters worse, the men were just as gorgeous in their sport coats and designer jeans. They also confidently wore pinks, pastels, and checkered plaid. It would take some getting used to— one doesn't see a lot of men sporting pastels in the Windy City.

I was fascinated by these women. I felt like a photographer for National Geographic tracking the graceful gazelle and watching in awe from the shadows, capturing every movement.

Eavesdropping on conversations, I didn't hear one "fuck." Not one, the entire time I was there. Really, *what the fuck?* I grew up as an Italian in Chicago. According to my mom, when I was about four years old, I was in the kitchen putting on my coat, getting ready to go out with a family friend. I was a big girl. I could put on my own coat. I put my arms through the sleeves of my faux fur coat and started to zip it up, but it got stuck. In a moment of sheer frustration, I unleased a slew of profanity that would have made a grown man blush. My poor mom had no idea what to do with this chubby-thighed little sweetheart in a ruffled dress dropping f-bombs. See, while other kids were watching wholesome shows like Ed McMahon's *Star Search*, I was at my grandma's eating manicotti and watching *The Godfather*, learning the ins and outs of the Corleone family.

There was a sophistication and intrigue about the people who passed by the window of the restaurant. As I pushed my Southern mashed taters loaded with gravy around my plate, all I could hear in my head was, *You'll NEVER fit in. You're too fat for the South.*

Just under six weeks until moving day—how the hell was I going to lose a hundred pounds by then?

Okay, not realistic. Maybe sixty? Ummm, okay, twenty pounds. Or how about ten pounds before we move? That will be a great jump-start and seems totally reasonable.

The math was the easy part. How would I make it happen, though? My husband and I ate out literally every day. We knew each other's orders at McDonald's, Taco Bell, Arby's, Portillo's— the list went on. We'd been together for so long our food routine was a science. Someone picked up food, we stuffed our faces, I passed out, he played video games, repeat.

Once I got home, I was going to throw EVERYTHING out. No more carbs or pop or ice cream or cheese...*Whoa, hold on, let's not get crazy. I'm keeping some cheese. It's a protein, so that's good for me, right?*

And let's face it, the big guy could stand to lose about a hundred pounds himself. We'll start using the gym membership we've been paying for for years. We'll run and bike and swim. We've got this.

Dirty thirty was going to be the best year of my life. And since I'd be starting my new diet in a few days, I decided I might as well indulge a little over the weekend. "Yes, waiter, I'll take the chips and salsa, tacos, rice and beans with extra sour cream and cheese, and then ice cream and cake please!"

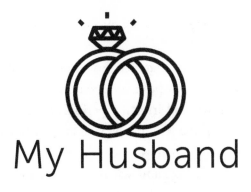

My Husband

I've never considered myself especially lucky in love. Rather, I've always felt like the character Gigi Phillips in the 2009 movie *He's Just Not That Into You*. (If you haven't seen it, drop everything and watch it now.) Like Gigi, I read more into every nice gesture, every kind word.

Growing up, I was always more into guys than they were into me. I felt pressure to find love, or something close to it, as it seemed to be happening for all my friends. In college, I set up my bestie (the shopper) with her now husband and they have two handsome boys. They loved each other the moment they met, and I envied that.

After college, I was optimistic about what the world had in store for me and felt ready to hit the real-world dating game: no more college dudes. I was confident that all the men I'd now meet would be mature. Boy was I wrong.

I'm not overly critical, but I don't consider how long you can hold a keg stand or how much weed you can smoke before passing out or puking solid metrics for determining a partner.

I was borderline insecure about my appearance at this point but hoped that my charming and funny personality would win over my dream guy. I'd put on a lot of weight in college—not the normal freshman fifteen but a whopping fifty pounds in less than six months. This came after being diagnosed with polycystic ovary syndrome (PCOS).

I would come to learn that PCOS was no joke and came with some super-awesome symptoms: extreme weight gain, excessive facial hair, infertility, and irregular periods. Most people experience different combinations of the side effects. Since I don't do anything half-assed, I had all the side effects to the max. Try feeling sexy in the dating game when you're worried about a five-o'clock shadow.

To help with the PCOS I took this awful medicine called metformin, whose primary purpose is to help diabetics regulate their sugar. I wasn't diabetic—my body just didn't know what to do with sugar. The medicine came with a 5 percent chance of making me sick. So, of course, it made me brutally sick. I sometimes missed classes because I was throwing up so much.

Over the years, I tried every diet, from the more well-known ones, such as Atkins and Weight Watchers (I mean, if it worked for Oprah…) and Jenny Craig, to the lesser-known "I've lost all hope and this needs to work" diets that involve only drinking broth, or only eating at a certain time of day, or only eating apples while standing on your head. If someone had invented it, I tried it. Each one worked for a while, but after I'd lost twenty or so pounds, the weight crept back on.

During this time, I went on crappy date after crappy date. This was a time before Tinder and Bumble. You couldn't just swipe left or right. Instead, you'd engage in long discussions on AOL Instant Messenger (look it up, kids) or on the phone for days, weeks, or months before meeting.

Technically, there were dating sites and yes, I did meet some gentlemen this way, including my future husband, but back then, if you met someone on the Internet, you never admitted that to anyone. You would be judged and warned about the dangers—about the perverts who lurked online.

You also never knew what to expect on your date, as photos were scarce, hard to see, and usually somewhat (like twenty years, in some cases) dated. It was a process! Dating now is so easy: you snap a few pics, upload them with a few clicks, and within minutes you're ready for love—or whatever. *wink wink

Back then, which wasn't actually that long ago, I'd drive to my local Walgreens, head to the back of the store to the vast and bustling photo section (there would be an actual line in the photo department), and scan my grainy pictures onto a CD to later be loaded onto my dating profile. It's a wonder that with all the hassle, online dating took off.

Then I'd sit and wait for someone to wink at me or send me a *hi*. I got a few winks and *hi*'s and went on a few dates, but old habits die hard. I continued to be the chaser and not the one being chased.

And then, one day, *he* sent me a *hi*.

I sent one back and a few days later we were at Chili's enjoying a dinner for two. This should probably have been my first clue that romance was going to be non-existent in the relationship. Look, there's nothing wrong with grabbing some baby back ribs with the family, but on a first date? C'mon. At least it wasn't Denny's, I guess.

As he walked through the door, I noticed he was taller than I'd expected, maybe six-foot-three or six-foot-four, but overall, he looked remarkably similar to his photos, so that was good. No surprises. He had a big teddy-bear-like frame, heavier on the top than the bottom, and was covered in tattoos. His tattoos weren't alarming—a sun, a Celtic cross, his family crest. Nothing that looked to have been inked in prison. I was in my "I want you to be a good guy who looks like a bad boy" phase. There aren't many of those guys out there.

He was nice and had kind blue eyes. And he seemed to be into me, so good enough.

For a few hours we ate and talked about our lives and our dreams for the future. I told him I was looking to build a career and not necessarily a family, and that I needed to make sure he was okay with someone who didn't have the desire to be a mom. Plus, with the damn PCOS who knew if I could even have kids.

I should have seen the red flag waving through the air: he had no goals. He was happy with the life of mediocrity he'd built. At the time, I saw him as someone who was settled, not looking for change, and that was something I could get behind—for the moment.

We said goodbye and then I didn't return his calls for almost two weeks.

Was this it? I wondered. Was this as good as it was going to get? We were like friends who'd always known each other, but there were no fireworks. Hell, there weren't even sparks. But I'd never felt butterflies or that pit in my stomach around any guy. I figured that was just something that happened in the movies or fairy tales.

So, we started dating. Well, in reality, we never really dated. In that critical time when romantic, fun activities and getting to know each other happens, we just sort of slid into a relationship. He never picked me up or held open the door for me. We were just in places together. Fairly quiet, he was happy to let me own the room. Our lifestyle was uneventful. Together, we were lazy. He treated me like one of the guys, and I acted like one. We would pee with the door open and complement each other on impressive burps. I certainly didn't feel like his hot, sexy girlfriend. I know we laughed a lot, but I can't remember a single conversation we ever had.

I continued to wonder: was it better to be in a relationship without spark with someone who was kind and funny and who loved you than to search for something that might never be?

Six months later, we moved in together. We were roommates and best friends. I always thought it was weird that we'd go months or even years without kissing or holding hands or, well, having sex. But we both struggled with low self-esteem, self-hatred, and weight issues, all of which played a major factor.

He was faithful, though. He always said he was too lazy to cheat. In a loveless, passionless marriage, it's often another woman who steals the man's fire away. In our case, her name was World of Warcraft (WoW), an online world where he was a hero. At home, I spent almost all my time alone. We actually met someone on our honeymoon who played WoW and that was all they talked about. It was the only thing he got excited about.

Once, I waited in the car for him for twenty minutes. I was picking him up and we were going out for dinner at, wait for it, Olive Garden. I thought he was getting ready, or in the bathroom—you know, something important. But he was finishing a quest. Yes, finishing a fucking quest while I sat and waited because he couldn't let down his online friends.

My loneliness led me to food, and I'd sleep out of boredom. I'd assumed I was just lazy.

So I was excited about a fresh start in North Carolina. It would all be different, right?

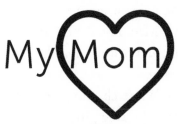

My Mom

"Mom, it's official! I got the promotion and I'm moving to North Carolina in six weeks…"

In my family, it's always been just the three of us: my mom, my baby brother, and me. We've always been close. To this day I call my brother "baby brother," even though he's only four years younger that I am and is now a chiropractor in Atlanta.

My favorite childhood moments involved laughing in the kitchen so hard we'd cry. When my mom and I have these laughing fits, we break into high-pitched squeals and aren't able to communicate like civilized people anymore. We've always understood each other and have a weird language all our own. She did everything for my brother and me. If we wanted to play a sport or stay late at school to make props for the play or take on a part-time job that required a vehicle, she made it happen. To this day I'm not sure how she did it. I get tired thinking about it.

For over twenty years she was a pack-a-day smoker. She was also slightly overweight and not athletic at all (don't throw a ball at her—it will just hit her in the head). But she was always inspiring me through her perseverance and hard work. My grandmother was exactly the same. I'm certain that my drive is an inherited trait. Three generations of badass, independent, strong, driven women. My grandma used to say, "If someone doesn't want to go with you to do something, piss on them and go alone."

One day, my mom decided to put down the cigarettes and get her ass on a treadmill. She barely made it two minutes the first time. This was the point where I would have given up and had a smoke and a Big Mac. But she didn't. She kept going, adding minutes and miles, and before long, she was completing her first 5k race—3.125 miles.

I stood on the sidelines cheering her on as she flew by with a big smile on her face. I was so proud in that moment but couldn't help but feel sad knowing that she was twenty-three years older than I was and accomplishing so much, and I was winded from walking and standing. Thirty-five minutes later she sprinted across the finish line grinning ear to ear.

Like the little girl walking around the house in her mom's too-big shoes and all her jewels, I wanted to be just like her. So, I got a gym membership and started doing laps on the track.

A few months later, I finished my first 5k. It was miserable. I was covered in sweat, I didn't smile, my legs hurt, and things were jiggling in places that shouldn't jiggle. But running right next to me was my mom, who would go on to become a two-time full and four-time half Ironman triathlete, cheering me on the whole time.

And so, calling my mom and telling her I was moving was heart-wrenching, but in true Mom fashion, she was supportive and even offered to help with the move, which was more than I could say for the man I was married to.

A few months went by, and I concluded that I officially hated North Carolina. I just wanted to go back home. I missed my mom. I missed our weekend shopping sprees and comparing receipts to see who'd gotten the best deals. I missed cuddling up on the couch with her to watch Lifetime movies (we've probably seen every Lifetime movie ever made). I also missed my friends. I was lonely.

And I was just as fat as ever, weighing the most I'd ever weighed in my life and wearing the second-largest-sized jeans from the plus-size store.

On social media, I posted photos that screamed "look how great my life is and how much fun I'm having." Inside, I was miserable and couldn't see a way out of this mental state.

Finally, one day, sitting in traffic with the top of my blue Volkswagen Bug convertible down, my hair whipping around in the wind, I lost it. I'm not sure what came over me in that moment—it was a release of months and years of unhappiness and disappointment in myself, and it all came rushing out in a flood of tears.

The only logical thing that came into my mind was *Call your mom.*

"Hi, Mom." *Sniffle, sniffle.*

"Dina, is that you? Hello?"

Sniffle, sniffle. "Yes, it's me."

"Honey, what's wrong? Did something happen? Are you okay?"

Loud, uncontrollable sobbing.

"Hello? Are you there?"

Unintelligible mumbling.

Finally, I blurted out, "I'm so sad!"

"What's wrong?" my mom asked again. "Are you okay?"

"I hate my life. I'm," *sniffle,* "so unhappy with myself, with my weight, my marriage. And I hate Raleigh."

I shocked her speechless. I knew I'd done a great job of hiding my feelings over the years. Then she started crying lightly as well. I knew she felt helpless and wished she could hug me.

After soothing me with some calming words, she said, "Honey, you should find a therapist to talk with. You have a lot of emotions and need someone who can properly help you."

A therapist? I thought. *How the hell is a therapist going to fix my problems? Maybe if they were formerly fat? Can I can search for that in their bios? Hmm...*

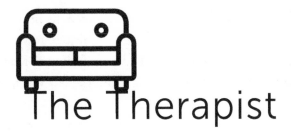

The Therapist

Nope, too stuffy looking. Nah, too young. No, no, no, all wrong.

Yes, I was judging books by their covers. I was looking online for a therapist who would get me. Not one who wore a suit and a condescending look. I needed someone I wouldn't feel insecure with. I pictured her wearing jeans, sneakers, and a dressy T-shirt. Her hair would be up in a messy ponytail and she'd wear just a hint of makeup. I wanted someone I could imagine sharing the tales of my life with over coffee or a burger. Someone who had a cool, casual demeanor. If I was going to give this a fair shot, I needed someone who would understand me and not judge me.

Next. Next. Let's mark her down as a maybe. Next…wait—who's this?

She was only about five to ten years older than I was, if I had to guess, originally from Minnesota (close enough to Chicago to consider her a Midwesterner, like me), and had a genuine, sincere face. Her eyes were as green as summer grass, she had fair skin spotted with a few freckles, and deep auburn hair that was wild and wavy. I immediately felt like I could trust her and tell her all my secrets.

I totally believe in signs when it comes to whether you're on the right track. As I nervously walked into the building where her office was for my first appointment, my guard up, I told myself,

Let's just see how this goes. It's not going to be easy—she's going to have to work for it.

She welcomed me warmly, and as she ushered me into her office, I was greeted by a huge canvas print of…Chicago. It was my sign; she was the right person for me. I had been feeling so alone, so far away from the place I loved so much, and there it was in front of me.

The hour flew by. During that time, I shared what would become the building blocks of a six-year relationship. After that first visit, I started seeing her every Thursday at 6:00 p.m., come hell or high water. We talked about everything: my childhood, my family, my weight, my husband, and all my sadness. She never judged, just listened and asked thought-provoking questions. She also never told me what to do. We worked through my life together, step-by-step, with her playing the role of an unbiased third-party angel.

One day, feeling chipper and confident, I walked into her office and said, "I'm regaining control of my life. I'm not going to feel this way any longer."

I'd been in North Carolina for a few years by this point, and not only had I not lost weight, I'd gained a lot. I barely recognized my face. My cheeks were so large my eyes looked almost shut. I wanted big, sexy Kardashian eyes, and I'd tried tons of makeup techniques to make my eyes look bigger, not realizing that until I lost the weight, it was counterproductive.

I'd also been doing my research about something else—I was seriously considering having gastric sleeve surgery. But I needed my trusty sign to know for sure if it was right for me.

My therapist and I mostly talked about how I needed to change my mind and not just my body, and we also discussed the toll this change in mindset would take on my marriage.

My marriage now revolved solely around food. Everything we

did was about food—it was the only way we communicated. My therapist warned me that I'd likely experience even more struggles in my rocky relationship if I started focusing on losing weight and changing my habits around food and he didn't, and she gave me several techniques I could use to help my marriage get through this new phase. But I wasn't even sure I wanted it to.

My husband and I had gone to marriage counseling, and that therapist had told us several times that we were great friends and that was how our marriage had survived all those years. I wanted to be married to my best friend, but I also needed love and romance. I wondered if we weren't intimate because he didn't find me attractive with all the extra weight. He would always say that he didn't want to be intimate because he wasn't happy about his own appearance, but then he'd shove cheeseburgers in his mouth, making me doubt that he had any desire to change. It was hard to process.

What I knew for certain was that I needed to focus on me and my journey. I'd always been a people pleaser, worried what others thought and concerned about their feelings rather than my own. I'd convinced myself I'd rather be unhappy than make someone else unhappy.

I told my therapist about how I'd sit in meetings at work and could focus only on how I barely fit in the chair. I assumed everyone was staring at my fat rolls as I pulled up to the table, that everyone was looking at every piece of candy I ate. I was careful about how much food I put on my plate in front of people, so they wouldn't see me eat like a fat person, but then I'd stop and get fast food on the way home to fill the void. Or I'd sneak candy from the vending machine in the kitchen—sometimes I'd buy two or three full-sized candy bars and binge-eat them in my office with the door closed. I also made jokes about the food I was eating, in the hopes it would stop others from doing it behind my back. People can be so cruel.

I shared with my therapist that every decision I made in my life started with me asking myself, "Will my weight be a factor in this activity?" I missed going to sporting events and plays with friends (the seats were too small); I was the purse holder when everyone went go-karting; I never went to the beach or on a boat or canoeing. I'd never traveled to Europe, since the flight was too long in those tiny seats. I let my weight determine my levels of fun, happiness, self-worth, and self-love.

I told her about how people cheered for me when I ran my 5k races. They'd shout, "You can do it," but what I heard was, "We're cheering for you because you're fat and you need extra encouragement because you might not finish." I always found the treadmill in the corner, or the yoga mat in the back. I hated the mirrors in all these classes because no matter how hard I tried to be invisible, there was a neon sign pointing to me that said: "Look here. Look. Look—is she kidding herself in this class?"

But a piece of advice my therapist gave me has stuck with me to this day, and I remember it any time I'm getting in my own head:

"In a moment of self-doubt, stop the thoughts and derail your thinking onto positive thoughts. Focus on something else: the lamp in the meeting, your weekend plans, your puggy." I always refer to my dog, a pug, as a puggy, he's just so darn cute. "Think of anything else until the feeling passes. Do this every time these negative thoughts creep in, even if you have to do it fifty times a day."

It doesn't matter how good I'm feeling about myself—insecurity will sometimes creep up. Recently, I sat on a panel for fearless women. I had accomplished so much to be proud of. But I sat next to Miss North Carolina. Yup, a real-life beauty queen. She was the picture of perfection: blonde wavy hair that grazed the middle of her back and swung gracefully as she walked, eyes as crystal blue as the most beautiful oceans, a toothpaste-commercial smile, flawless skin—even her damn nails were perfect. She was like Barbie come to life.

And there I was (in my own mind, not reality), a dumpy brunette with bad skin, fat thighs, and saggy boobs. In truth, I looked great. My weight was good, my hair was on point, and my makeup was flawless. And I realized I needed to stop and remember what my therapist had said all those years earlier.

After that meeting with my therapist, the next time I was in a meeting that could have easily been an email, sitting there with the candy dish staring me down, I paid attention to the thoughts: *You're too fat for this chair. Your rolls are hanging over this chair.* And then I told them to stop. And I focused on the lamp on the table. *How long has it been there? Is it from another part of the building? Why is my fat sticking out the side of the chair? No, back to the lamp. Is it brass? What would happen if I moved it? Would anyone notice? How much did it cost? How tall is it in centimeters? Is it heavy?* Then my mind headed back to the meeting. "Blah blah blah, something about human resources, blah blah, meeting dismissed." I made it through almost the entire meeting not thinking about the chair.

As the months passed, I continued to apply this technique and noticed negative thoughts popping up less and less—until one awful day. I was sitting in the top section of a college auditorium listening to a company town hall. The seat was a tight squeeze, to say the least. The chair's bolt dug into the side of my leg. It hurt so much that soon, the pain was all I could think of. It felt as if knives were jabbing me over and over. I tried so hard to focus on the room, a lamp, the stage—anything to get my mind off the pain. When the meeting was over, I headed to the bathroom and saw that my leg was bloody and bruised. I'd been telling myself I needed a definitive sign about getting the gastric sleeve surgery.

At that moment, I made my decision. My bruised, bloody leg was my sign.

I needed to start my journey to freedom: Freedom from the fear in which I lived my life. Freedom to go and do what I wanted. Freedom to become who I deserved to be.

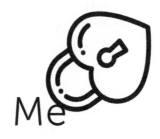

Me

It was my favorite time of year again. Fall was in the air, and all I could think of was pumpkin spice: pumpkin spice lattes, candles, soap, lotion, waffles, cereal, tea—all things pumpkin spice. Oh, and sweaters and boots and bonfires and flannels. Seriously my favorite time of year.

And there I sat in my big house, all alone. No dinner with my husband to celebrate the new me. He wasn't there. Just me, surrounded by my final junk-food meal: a Big Mac, a cheeseburger, large fries (I did share a few with my puggy), a chocolate shake, and two soft, warm chocolate chip cookies. Yup, all in one sitting. I got sick to my stomach but wanted to get all the tastes in.

I'd been eating my favorites excessively for the last week—ice cream (that I would eat by scooping it with chocolate wafers), extra, extra cheesy pizza, and tacos (my favorite food group) from my favorite local Mexican restaurant, Los Tres Amigos. I don't speak Spanish, but I'm pretty sure that meant "Best Fucking Tacos Ever."

I acted as if eating were an Olympic sport and I was trying to win a gold medal. I couldn't blame McDonald's or Los Tres Amigos. I lacked self-control.

I've always loved food, even though I'm a picky eater. As a child, I was praised by my Italian grandmother for not only finishing my plate full of food but for asking for seconds. How could something you're being praised for be bad?

Though I was never "thin" in the traditional sense, I wasn't overweight until the age of eighteen. I didn't hate my body until I started packing on the pounds in college. Even then, I still thought I looked good and had a pretty face. My self-image got flipped upside down in my sophomore year of college, at my boyfriend's frat house. During a party, he poked my stomach and said "big fat belly" in front of twenty-plus people. I went home that night and ate candy until I made myself ill. My bestie never left my side as I vomited.

That night triggered a chain reaction of decisions that led to years of self-abuse (a back and forth of binge-eating and radical diets) and, well, self-hate. It's amazing how someone can say something that they forget in the next moment but that you end up carrying with you for the rest of your life. How could anyone really love me when I looked the way I did? I wondered.

Tomorrow is the day, I thought, as I finished that final meal before embarking on a two-week, liquid, pre-surgery diet. *Tomorrow my life will change forever. Tomorrow will be a new beginning. Tomorrow will be about me and only me. No more letting others' words and actions dictate my happiness or my choices.*

At the hospital, the nurse was shocked that I was so fat but so healthy. She kept saying, "You're *sure* you're not on any meds?" No, I'm not on any meds. "But with your weight, do you have sleep apnea?" I responded no to every question. She was puzzled.

I put on my jumbo hospital gown and fuzzy socks and lay there, nervous and excited, waiting for my surgeon to arrive. He was handsome: fit and tall with strawberry blond hair (which I normally didn't find attractive—I like my men with dark hair, maybe salt-and-pepper, think smoldering, like Richard Gere in *Pretty Woman*). But more importantly, he was warm and caring. I trusted him and knew he believed in me and my journey.

I wondered what his wife looked like and assumed she was beautiful and thin. I mean, his job was to make fat people thin—could he ever love someone who looked like me?

These were the kinds of thoughts I'd been trying not to focus on.

As the anesthesia kicked in, I looked at my surgeon, who was calm and smiling, and drifted off counting backward and thinking about his wife.

"Ten." *I wonder if she's tall.*

"Nine." *I wonder if she's athletic.*

"Eight." *Does she have a career?*

"Seven." ...

"It's okay, Dina. You're safe, you're in the recovery room, and everything went great."

I'd woken up swinging like Rocky ready to fight Apollo Creed. I was so cold that I was shaking and my teeth were chattering. I felt as if I'd been dropped into ten feet of snow naked.

"Get her some more blankets. Hey, Dina, you're okay. We've got you."

After the nurses dodged my left hook for several moments, I started to come to. My surroundings came into focus.

Ok, I'm at the hospital. I haven't died. I'm alive and well. And sore.

I was also hungry. For the last two weeks I'd been on a gross, liquid diet. I just wanted a popsicle. My surgeon had said that after the surgery, I could have small amounts of water, broth, and Jell-O, and that once I could eat a whole popsicle and keep it down, I could go home. All I could think in that moment was *I want that fucking popsicle now!*

I drifted in and out of sleep over the next day. When I was awake, I walked to avoid blood clots, sipped my broth (yum), and watched the trashy daytime TV that I never got to watch.

Mostly, I was there alone, even though my husband had taken time off work "to care for me." He was filled with excuses about where he was and what he was doing.

According to the book *The Five Love Languages* by Gary Chapman, at our core, each of us prefers to give and receive love in a particular way. The languages are words of affirmation, acts of service, receiving gifts, quality time, and physical touch. What's important is to respect and nurture your partner's love language. My husband had never understood my love languages: quality time and physical touch. All I wanted was for him to be by my side, holding my hand. Instead, he would buy me gifts and flowers (his love language was gifts). I didn't want the fucking flowers—I wanted him to be there. When I was released from the hospital and ready to go home, he was nowhere to be found. Strike 1,000!

I spent the next few weeks on the couch recovering with my puggy by my side. Friends stopped by to go on little walks with me or sit with me, but my husband was noticeably missing from the picture. I didn't let it get me down—I let it fuel my fire. Every day I walked a little farther, a little faster, and a little longer, and before I knew it, two weeks had flown by and I was off to work.

The clothes that I'd once barely been able to button up were a little loose. Which was good because I was still healing, so I needed something comfy, but I also didn't want to look like I'd just rolled out of bed.

It wasn't easy being back at work, where there was a soda fountain (free) and candy everywhere I looked. Within my first week back there were two birthday cakes, one ice cream social, and a team lunch. I held strong; I hadn't gone through all that work for nothing. I *would not* sabotage myself this time. In the difficult moments, I thought about my bloody and bruised leg, about missing out on so many things, and about the sadness. I had to be strong—something I never felt I'd been.

Halloween and Thanksgiving came and went and then it happened: I hit my first goal. I'd lost seventy-five pounds. My reward was a pair of shiny black leather Tory Burch flats with a big gold emblem on the toe. Why Tory Burch flats? Because I hadn't been able to fit into them before. My feet had been too wide. They were the first of many rewards I gave myself for my progress.

As the weight continued to drop, my confidence rose. At 130 pounds lost, I felt as if I owned the world. It's a strange feeling, losing so much weight. I kept thinking, *Am I done? Is this my goal weight?* Having been about 150 pounds overweight for so many years, my goal weight just seemed like a made-up number. It wasn't real. I had never before believed I could be at that weight.

I was taking everything my surgeon had said as gospel. I ate how, when, and what I was supposed to, and I also followed a vigorous workout routine. At this point, I was training for my first half marathon. My mom and my other bestie (not the shopper but the CrossFit trainer/runner) would be running with me, by my side for every step. My mom had come up with this idea that every time I hit a mile marker, I should say out loud something I hadn't been able to do or hadn't felt comfortable doing in my heavier body.

And so I did.

Mile 1: "Run a half marathon."

Mile 2: "Drive a go-kart."

Mile 3: "Fit into the regular seat belts on a plane."

Mile 4: "Shop at the regular stores."

Mile 5: "Walk upstairs without getting winded."

Mile 6: "Fit in chairs or booths at restaurants."
Mile 7: "Go out dancing."
Mile 8: "Go swimming."
Mile 9: "Love myself."
Mile 10: "Wear heels and skinny jeans." (I still hate them both.)
Mile 11: "Be comfortable in the front of the room in yoga class."
Mile 12: "Believe in myself."
Mile 13: "Know that I am enough."

As I trained, the weight almost literally fell off. In meetings, I was able to focus on the topic and not my fat rolls. I had more energy, too. I was waking up earlier, going to bed later, and not wanting to sit around the house. I wanted to be out and about, shopping, and enjoying time with friends.

And in that time of pure joy and happiness, I gave my relationship of almost twelve years one last shot. I needed to give the marriage a fighting chance. I told myself that if he showed any effort, even just a little, I would go all in. I would fight for this to work.

I filled the bathroom with candles, put on romantic music, dimmed the lights, and turned on the shower. Then I walked out to the living room in just a towel and asked my husband to join me in the shower.

He looked up at me, unimpressed, and said, "I'm finishing a quest, give me a minute." I waited in that shower for what felt like hours. He never came.

As a single tear trickled down my face, I blew out each candle one by one. I turned off the music with my pruney fingers, put on an old T-shirt and sweatpants, grabbed my puggy, and went to bed. When he came in, two hours later, I lay there pretending to be asleep, my face turned into the pillow to muffle the sounds of my crying. I felt only rejection.

The next day, I asked for a divorce.

Part Two:
Grit and Moxie

She is unshakable not because she doesn't know pain or failure, but because she always pushes through. Because she always shows up and never gives up. Because she believes anything is possible no matter the odds.

www.bryananthonys.com

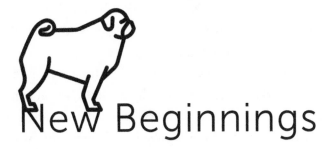# New Beginnings

Rage and determination will get you far in life.

I carried the damn minifridge from my husband's man cave on my back down sixteen stairs like the fucking Hulk. I sat on the floor of our home's lower level with a wood marker and colored in every nick and scratch. I patched every hole in the wall from pictures and art we'd collected over the years (weirdly, there were no pictures of us). And I packed up and prepped for sale the entire 3,400-square-foot house (which included four bedrooms, four bathrooms, an office, the man cave, a loft with a pool table, a kitchen, a dining room, a living room, and a foyer). All by myself.

We had built this "dream" home only three years prior—our version of having a baby to save the marriage. It was located in the gorgeous subdivision of Wake Forest, just outside Raleigh. Just ten years earlier, there had been nothing here but country roads and farmland. It was the kind of subdivision I would drive past and think, *Who lives there? What is their life like? What do they do for a living? Do they have a happy marriage and kids running around?* I imagined these people's perfect lives in their perfect homes.

And so, when my husband and I decided to build there, I'd painstakingly picked out every detail, wanting everything to be perfect. It didn't help that our builder's design center was five minutes away from my work. As you can imagine, this was where

I spent most of my lunch hours. It got to the point where everyone there knew me when I walked in. Dark cabinets? White? Rustic? Modern? Every decision needed to be right. And when the day came and I had to pick the final design, I was ready.

The cabinets were a dark walnut, and I chose cream and gray granite that sparkled in just the right light, almost as if it contained little flecks of glitter (glitter is my favorite color, besides pink, of course). The dark wood floors highlighted the two-story stone fireplace, above which the TV hung neatly. I was adamant about not wanting to see a single wire in the house. The tub in the master bathroom could have been confused for a pool it was so big. I'm not much for baths, which is weird given that I once owned a bath and body company, but my husband had demanded a tub big enough for his large frame, as he was a bath guy.

All my painstaking work paid off. It looked like a model home, something right out of a Pottery Barn catalog (I mean, I did get most of the furnishings from there). And when the time came, the house sold in a day and a half, only slightly under the asking price (which was the number we'd wanted in the first place). The new owners bought most of our furniture as well.

For us, this masterpiece had been a Band-Aid on an unhappy life.

For the first time ever, at thirty-five years old, I was going to create the life I'd always imagined. And for the first time in my entire life, I was going to live alone. I had gone from my mom's house to a dorm to a house with one bathroom and four roommates, and then back to my mom's house before moving in with my husband.

Now, it would just be me and the puggy. No roommates, no husband. It felt like freedom.

I found the perfect apartment, only a few years old, in an area of Raleigh called Cameron Village. It was perfect—only two and a half miles from work and just a few minutes from downtown Raleigh. To this day, it's still my favorite place to live in all of North Carolina. If I win the lottery, I'm going to buy a sweet little 1950s bungalow and spend my days rehabbing it (or at least overseeing the crew rehabbing it). This area is so expensive that a 1,200-square-foot bungalow without a garage and sometimes not even a driveway ranges from $350,000 to $800,000.

On any given day, I'd put on cute workout pants and a shirt with a positive message, such as "Go the extra mile, it's never crowded," or "Under construction" (this one confused a ton of people, as they thought I was announcing a pregnancy—um, I don't believe in Immaculate Conception, so that shirt went to Goodwill). Then I'd walk across the street to Flywheel to take a class with my favorite instructor. She led a class on Tuesdays that featured explicit rap music, creating the perfect trifecta for me: spin class, swearing, and rap. Count me in.

I became a regular at the local Starbucks and would meet friends for lunch or drinks. I shopped. A lot. I'd get manis and pedis.

The puggy and I would often go for leisurely strolls in the neighborhood, and he became a bit of a local celeb. One day, we were walking a few blocks from my apartment when a woman approached and asked if she could pet my puggy. "Sure," I said. "This is Bean."

"OMG," she replied. "I've heard about him from my friends who live in the area. Can I get a picture with him?"

I tried to play it cool as I said yes, but I'm sure I was grinning like an idiot.

Feeling great about how my life was going, I decided to jump into the dating pool. I was looking for someone who would respect my love languages, someone who had dreams and ambitions, someone who worked hard and didn't play games, and someone fit-ish—I didn't want some hunk who showed off his six-pack, but I did want someone who was in shape. After all, fitness had become an important part of my life.

Knowing that the attractive women of Raleigh, well poised in their seduction, would now be my dating competition, my insecurity flag flew high. But I didn't let it stop me or slow me down.

I got online and created a profile.

I'm a woman looking for a man. I'm 5'6". Okay, I'm really 5'5" ¾, but the ¾ is very important—short girls know what I'm saying—so I rounded up.

Curvy…no, athletic…no, average…no, curvy. Let's go with curvy. It was hard to turn off my "fat girl" brain.

Brown hair, brown eyes, divorced. Well, separated and waiting on those papers—in North Carolina you have to have separate residences for at least a year before you can file for divorce. After that, the process can take another two or three months if you agree on everything.

Likes? Hmmm, this would be more helpful if they had a drop-down box. Okay, I like Flywheel, my puggy, live music, movies in the park… What else? I'll come back to this later.

Ideal guy? Can I just say Ross from Friends (except the whole "we were on a break" thing) was handsome but not drop-dead gorgeous, approachable, smart, had a great career, and was funny. Perfect. I wanted someone who thought I was awesome. Someone who would stand up and say, "That's my girl!"

Okay, next sections. Do you have kids? Nope. Do you want them? Nope. That ship has sailed. I couldn't imagine starting at thirty-five years old. I know a lot of women do it, but I was set in my ways.

Okay, picture time. Something smiley. Everyone says that I have a great smile and the infamous "pretty face." I hated that. Couldn't I just be pretty and leave it at that? *Um, how about one that shows the pink, purple, and green highlights in my hair? One with the puggy because if they don't like pugs, they're OUT!*

Good enough. Now I post and wait…

The dating game had changed a lot in the last twelve years. I was instantly bombarded with messages.

All right then, let's check this out.

Bob1224 – "You're hot. Looking to hook up?"

Nope, delete.

SmoothSailor86 – "No kids? I can put a baby in you." *Nope*, delete.

MrCasanova22 – Dick pic.

Really? C'mon! Am I the kind of girl whose picture screams, "Please send pics of your dick, stat?" Is any girl's, for that matter? Is that even your dick?

Sixpack01 – "Hey, sexy."

Nope, delete.

Ladiesman1001 – "Wow, you're hot. You make me want to touch myself."

Who raised these morons? Where are their mothers?

And on and on. *Nope*, delete. *Nope*, delete. *Nope*, delete.

A few made it through and they contributed to what would end up being an interesting dating life. There was bowling with the software guy (who made me pay the nine dollars for my lane and shoes); an awful dinner with the PR guy (I would have rather gnawed my arm off than see him again); Mexican food with the HR guy (who kept banging his hands on the table and saying, "What else can I tell you about me?"); canoeing with the lawyer (not bad, but man did he like to talk about himself—oh and get this, I "didn't ask enough questions about him"); drinks and s'mores with the insurance guy (insurance is so boring); Mediterranean food with the architect (at least the food was good); drinks at a brewery with the sales guy…

Nope, nope, nope. I suffered through thirty-eight first dates, and only a handful of men made it to the second date. One made it to the third.

After weeding through hundreds of crappy messages and dick pics, this was what I'd ended up with—a sea of semi-attractive, boring, self-absorbed men with dad bods.

That's it, I'm destined to be alone.

Thinking back to my first weekend in Raleigh, when I'd thought all the guys were perfect, I wondered if my standards had gone up or if I'd been drunk that night.

Wait, who's this?

@Him1976 – "Hi, hope you're having a nice day. Cubs or Soxs?"

He was forty-four, originally from Florida but had spent ten years in Chicago, a dad of two teenagers, wasn't living at home, attractive in his picture, and his opening line was perfect.

"I'm not a big baseball fan, so go Bears!"

Cue the adorable, sexy banter.

Him

Ba-boom, ba-boom. My heart was racing about a thousand miles an hour, my hands were sweating and shaking, and a warm feeling was rushing through my body.

It was him.

And he was even more attractive in person than he was in his dating profile and on FaceTime. Tired of crappy dates, I'd started using FaceTime to chat before committing to anything, even a coffee. On FaceTime, I could tell right away if there were sparks or red flags (one guy didn't fully grasp the concept and turned off his camera but forgot to mute his mic and started peeing while we were chatting).

It was him, sauntering toward me.

He was tall, about 6'2", had lush, salt-and-pepper hair I was dying to run my hands through, a perfectly kept beard with just a few streaks of gray, a natural tan from working outside, and a toned body. I wondered what was under his formfitting shirt—maybe a six-pack? All I knew was I wanted to know more. He also had a perfect ass in his jeans and seemed to be one of the few men in his mid-forties who understood how horrible dad jeans were. His eyes were a light shade of brown, not quite hazel, and I knew they held secrets. He had a scar next to his left eye, and his hands were slightly callused—he was a man who knew what hard work was.

He was the most gorgeous man I'd ever seen, and he was on a date with me.

I was hooked that very moment.

As the musician played, we ate, we drank, we laughed (sometimes a little too loudly for the musician's friends). At one point I glanced down at my phone only to realize that three and a half hours had flown by. I've tried to remember what we talked about that night, but all I can remember is that it felt right.

We took a stroll through the area, which was filled with restaurants and bars and cute shops. Strings of lights hung from the trees whispered romance. My black cotton wrap dress fluttered and danced in the slight breeze that accompanies late-summer nights. All the stars were out, and the temperature was just cool enough that I needed my jean jacket—thank god, because on most North Carolina summer nights, I was a big sweaty mess. Here, I usually just sweat from May until October with no break. I was in the best shape of my life. I looked great. I felt amazing.

And then he kissed me, and my heart felt as if it were going to jump out of my chest. As we wrapped up the evening, he asked for a second date, and after another passionate but not overzealous kiss, we went our separate ways.

I think I'm in love!

My heart had NEVER felt this way. It was magical. I could hear birds chirping. I felt as though I were in a Disney movie. *Move over, Cinderella, it's my turn!* I was thirty-five years old, and for the first time in my life, I was feeling those butterflies.

A day passed. And another. And another. And another. And finally, the day before our next date, in the semi-late evening, my phone pinged.

"Hi, I hope you had a great day. Looking forward to our date tomorrow."

Holy crap, it's him. I jumped up and down. *It's him. He hasn't forgotten me.* I broke out into the "it's him" dance, shaking my booty: *It's him, it's him, it's him!*

I figured I'd been ghosted and the day prior had sworn off all men. *Okay, men are back on, the date is back on. Houston, we're good to go.*

A few dates later, wanting to kick up the romance, I invited him for dinner on the roof of my apartment building. I'd been recently promoted, was living a pretty swanky, glamorous life at this point, in my six-story apartment where a two-bedroom cost more than most people's mortgages. The building overlooked the downtown skyline, and the roof was lined with strings of Edison bulbs. With just a click of a remote, I started the outdoor fireplace, which crackled in the light breeze. I'd ordered fancy-pants pizza from the restaurant across the street and had cracked open a bottle of pinot grigio.

In that moment, I couldn't believe this was my life. I was one of the thin, beautiful Raleigh girls I'd stared at and envied, and I was having a romantic dinner with this stunning man. In my mind, he was perfect.

But he was guarded and mysterious. Even though I could tell he liked me, I was determined to play it cool and not fall into old patterns. I didn't want to get in deep and then find out he "just wasn't that into me." I resisted all the negative thoughts in my head, and I wouldn't let myself check his dating profile to see when he was last online—I was going to let love take me on this journey. If it was meant to be, it would be. But a little help from Ed Sheeran wouldn't hurt.

Ed Sheeran was coming to Raleigh, and I had a pair of floor-seat tickets. I'd been trying to decide who to take, and then it dawned on me: *ask him.*

Should I ask him? What if he says no? At least I'll know where I stand. And there's a chance he'll say yes.

I started typing: "Hey, what's up?" *That's stupid.* Erased it. "Hi, I was hoping you would accompany me to the Ed Sheeran concert next week. I have two tickets." *What the hell was that? When have I ever used the word "accompany"?* Tried again. "Hey, I have two tickets to Ed Sheeran—wanna go with me?"

I sent it. Then I waited. Waited. Waited.

We'd been dating for a few months but hadn't yet had the "are we exclusive" conversation. I hadn't wanted to bring it up and scare him away.

Maybe he's at work, or out with friends, or taking a nap, or on a date. OMG, what if he's on a date and I'm gushing about my stupid concert tickets and am about to be rejected? I'll have to go by myself to the most romantic concert ever and spend my whole life alone in my fabulous apartment, just me and my puggy.

Ping. "Sure, that sounds fun."

I repeated his words out loud. *Sure, that sounds fun. He said yes! Hmmm, wait. "Sure, that sounds fun," could mean "I have nothing better to do next Saturday night," or "This could be the greatest night ever."*

Okay, reel in the crazy. He said yes. That's all that matters.

The logical next steps were as follows: get a new top and book appointments for a blowout, a makeover, a manicure, a pedicure, and an eyebrow and bikini wax. After all, it was going to be the best night of my life. I had to look the part.

To find the perfect top, I went to just about every store in the mall and scoured every inch of the Internet—I wanted something black, something not obviously sexy but sophisticated sexy, and something that showed a little shoulder. Since I'd lost weight, my clavicle bone had become my best feature, so I wanted to flaunt it.

I already had the perfect pair of pants to wear with my new top: my fitted dark JLO jeans with white stitching down the legs and on the pockets. If anyone understands a woman with curves and a little extra booty, it's JLO. I looked like a million dollars in those jeans. These were also my smallest pair of jeans, so mentality wise, wearing them felt awesome. Flywheel four or five times per week was paying off.

Since they were a little long for flats, I paired them with my TOMS wedges. These were no ordinary wedges: they had a sweet crisscross at the toe that showed off my freshly pedicured toes and wrapped around the ankle to create a sexy silhouette. The best part was they add three inches to my height, making me a very sexy 5'8" and ¾.

When I felt I'd exhausted all options in terms of finding an adorable shirt and had made peace with the fact that I would be going to see Ed Sheeran with the sexiest man I'd ever dated in a black, flowy, hefty garbage sack, the dating and shopping gods suddenly merged forces and said to me, "Try this one last store." With my excitement level at a two and feeling defeated, I walked through the door. There it was—a flowy black racerback top with the thinnest of straps and some ruffles at the waist. A little naughty and a little nice.

In the fitting room, I said, "Please, God, I don't ask for much, and, well, just let this shirt fit and look good and I'll owe you one." And, just like that, my prayers were answered. It fit like a glove, as if it were custom made for my body! God does work in mysterious ways.

The big night arrived. "Let's grab a glass of wine before heading to our seats," he said with a smile. In that moment, I knew I was in for a great night.

We made our way to our seats to find that there would be only twenty rows between us and my favorite singer, Ed. Or, as I like to call him, Eddie. He looks more like an Eddie. Ed seems too serious.

"Hello, Raleigh!" Eddie said, walking onto the stage. "Are you ready for the best night ever?"

You read my mind, Eddie!

As he played "Dive," my favorite song, I sang my heart out—off key, of course—and meant every word. And the man I'd been crazy about for the last three months looked at me and said, "You're the most beautiful woman here. I could see myself loving you one day."

Holy shit, Christian Grey—it's about to get little Fifty Shades in here!

When we got back to my place, we lay in bed cuddling for what felt like hours, his arm tucked under my head. We were like two puzzles pieces that just fit together. It was happening. I'd finally found my heart.

In true whirlwind-romance fashion, we met in July, fell in love in September (with a little help from Eddie), and took a weekend trip in October to meet his family in Virginia Beach. Seeing the bond he had with them made me love him more. I wanted to be part of his world so badly. My birthday also fell on that weekend, and I woke up that morning to the most perfect card—"Happy Birthday. I'm the luckiest man alive"—and a dozen pink roses next to the bed. I couldn't believe that only six years from the lowest point of my life and my thirtieth birthday, this was my life.

In December, he became my nurse and caregiver after I had a tummy tuck, my treat to myself for four years of hard work losing weight and keeping it off. The surgeon removed sixteen pounds of extra skin and fat.

My new man doted on me and changed my bandages, which

was a gross job. He was my angel. Little did I know there was a devil lurking within his secretive eyes. Given how many Lifetime movies I've watched, you'd think I would have seen the signs. But I was completely blind, living in this perfect bubble I'd created for us.

Our fairytale continued, though. In February, we moved in together. I didn't want to wait. I was happy, truly happy, for the first time in my life. He made dinner every night, and even if he just made grilled cheese it felt like a feast (especially since he'd cook with nothing under his apron). He was passionate, and I simply loved being with him. I had to refrain from telling him I loved him a million times a day. He'd tell me I was beautiful and he didn't deserve me and all I could think was *I want to marry this man; I want to have and hold him for sicker or poorer for the rest of my life; I want him to make me grilled cheese sandwiches, naked, until we're eighty.*

I was living in this parallel universe where someone wanted to take care of me. This was new to me.

We also shared responsibilities. When he did the dishes, I did the laundry, and then we'd fold clothes together in front of the TV. I'd get up in the morning and make his coffee and toast then pack our lunches. I wanted to do it—it's crazy how much more you give when you feel appreciated. It was difficult to get used to, since I'd spent twelve years waiting on my ex hand and foot and cleaning up after him, even though I'd been working just as many hours as he had.

Was this what all "real" relationships were like? Had I wasted twelve years settling when I could have been happy? Or was this just my person, my soulmate? Had I needed to live my other life to be able to see all the love that was out there?

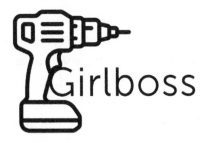

Girlboss

Have you ever had so many ideas in your head you feel it might explode? My brain runs about a thousand miles a minute. At my core I'm a creator and an innovator. People often say to me, "This is great, you should make it a business."

In the midst of my relationship bliss, I started daydreaming about my days as an entrepreneur, and my inner girlboss and innovator began gnawing at me.

Remember that little bath-bomb cupcake company that I started at twenty-four? Delish Gourmet Bath Bakery, my first entrepreneurial adventure. Back then, I was bolder, not afraid to take chances and risk it all. I also didn't have much to lose. I lived on ramen, and not the fancy ramen that's popping up in restaurants everywhere but the twenty-nine-cent ramen. When I had a great week, I'd splurge and get the seventy-cent version.

This fearlessness was sometimes overshadowed by self-doubt though—how could I be smart enough to start a business? I mean, my minor in college was business and I finished with a D average.

Even back then, I knew that I didn't know everything, but I did know I needed a mentor I could trust and who would have my best interests at heart. I started to think of the type of mentor who would be right for me. Since I had the creative side down, I needed a business genius, someone who'd been around the block and would be patient with me.

The mentor I found is someone I now love like a father. He just happened to be a fancy-pants VP of sales for a big company. He had great feedback for me on my business plan, and our generic meetings transformed into planning sessions and time spent creating business-growth objectives. I would listen in awe, trying to soak up every word like a sponge. He loved to give me advice while he was sweeping up the shop—and with all the bath-bomb powder, sweeping was always necessary! He'd grab the broom and transform into Zig Ziglar.

Back then, we decided that to make a splash, I needed to go big. The next logical next step was to take my little bath-bomb cupcakes to the Chicago Merchandise Mart for what is now the Chicago Gift Market: three days, hundreds of brands, and thousands of buyers, which included boutique owners and name-brand stores. The booth was expensive, a little over three thousand dollars, but the organizers were sweet and let me split up the payments. Other companies were spending thousands if not tens of thousands on their booth spaces.

My mom and I showed up with our two hundred dollars' worth of decorations from TJ Maxx and Home Goods. I was embarrassed to be putting together this home-grown booth but knew that my mentor and my mom would both be disappointed in me if I didn't give it my all. Hell, I'd be disappointed in me. So, I put on my big-girl panties and rocked it out. I spent the next three days talking to anyone who would listen about what a bath-bomb cupcake was and why they needed it in their shop.

In those three days, we signed 150 boutiques and the online division of Bath and Body Works (that's a whole other book in the making). It was the best experience of my life, and I'd never worked harder. Ours was the busiest booth at the show. The hand-crafted bath treats were created by my army of makers and me. Each one was packed into a cupcake mold, and the bubble-bath frosting was made from scratch and piped on just like in a real bakery.

One of my favorites was Birthday Cake, which had the most delicious smell. If you closed your eyes, you could almost hear people singing "Happy Birthday." The bright yellow "cake" was frosted with the richest white icing and topped with pastel sprinkles. Simple and sweet.

Now, working in my corporate gig, I was feeling the pull to do something creative again. I wanted to teach others that they could do anything they put their minds to. I also wanted to create something with him—to build a business and a life with him. And, well, getting away from the corporate bullshit would be icing on the cake.

I'd built an amazing career that paid well and came with great benefits, vacation days, and a 401K—and I wanted to leave it all behind and gamble on me. I'd spent the last ten years in the corporate grind working to make other people money, to make other people happy, to build other people's success. Don't get me wrong—corporate wasn't all bad. I'd picked up a couple of neat tricks along the way. I was just craving something different.

One date night, he looked at me and said, "Let's create a business that combines the best of both of us." The next day, my initial idea was born. My business would not only inspire others to tap into their creative side but would also give them a space to do the creation—and he would help me build it.

A master woodworker, he had immense talent. Everything he built was precise and well-made. His brain worked just like mine—he would see it and then create it and it would be perfect.

He taught me how to check the wood at Home Depot to make sure it was straight, how to measure and line up the wood for a correct cut every time, and how to use a saw. Yup, I use power tools. I know, it's pretty badass.

We laid every piece of flooring together. Well, he laid it, but I was the hander, and that job is just as important. He built and painted every table, and I built the fixtures—have you ever put together ten large bookcases from IKEA? I'm pretty sure I speak Swedish now. I created our logo and styled the studio. It was back-breaking, exhausting work, but we did it together, no arguments. We were the perfect team.

When the studio was done, I couldn't believe my vision had come to life. Our space was nestled between a dry cleaner's shop and boxing gym. Pulling into the parking lot, visitors would be greeted by an illuminated white sign that proudly displayed the business name: KNACK. The large front window was adorned with *KNACK DIY Craft Studio* and the logo, and it lent so much brightness and warmth to the space. The floors were a red-brown mahogany with tiny grooves, creating an upscale rustic look (the material was actually the cheapest one Home Depot sold, but people were constantly complimenting it). The walls were bright white, and project kits added a splash of color (hell, we were the only spot in North Carolina where you could make your own nail polish!)

The projects on the walls featured wood signs that showed off his construction skills and my design and painting skills. One shelf displayed my famous bath-bomb cupcakes along with mini fairy gardens (yes, they were as cute as they sound).

The white tables were the perfect height to create while standing, or visitors could sit on our signature mint-green metal stools. There were hints of mint, our brand color, all over the studio.

My favorite part of the space was the photo wall, which was lined with 180 paint brushes that we had hand-dipped in mint-colored paint, and dried. It was a long and tedious project but made the shop.

As I said my goodbyes at my corporate job, it finally hit me: it was all up to me. I was once again about to embark on the scariest journey of all—entrepreneurship. But with my him and my family by my side, I knew I could tackle anything.

The grand opening was a hit. My mentor and family flew in to celebrate, and people came in waves to check out the new kid in town. People immersed themselves in little projects (painting acrylic keychains and creating baby succulent gardens with the most adorable painted pots). They remarked on the beautiful space and welcomed us to the community with open arms.

And then, on our official first day…crickets.

Is that an actual cricket walking across the floor? Where are the droves of people? They should be beating down the door to book classes! Don't they see what we have to offer? We're the DIY experts.

Maybe we'll have a better turnout tomorrow.

Tomorrow turned into a week and then two, and I realized that if I didn't put on my #girlboss thinking cap, I was going to be out of business before getting started.

I had a pep talk with myself and decided to do what I do best: innovate. I'd built a concept that was unique but had missed the mark and incorporated an old way of thinking—booking classes and workshops was so "been there, done that." And so, I ran a new plan past my mentor, my mom, and him: we would become the first DIY craft studio at which you create any time. Instead of signing up for a class, you could just come on in. You wouldn't have to wait for a date and time and then paint a stupid peacock you'd never hang in your house anyway.

I also created more projects; I think I have about nine thousand pins on Pinterest. I had inspiration coming out the wazoo but had to consider several factors—could someone else build the project, how long would it take, and how much would it cost. Surprisingly, in the world of DIY, once you start buying wholesale, most of the business costs are in the payroll and rent, not the projects.

Since there were no customers in the shop, I revamped the layout so that when people walked in, they could check out all the projects, which were perfectly presented on the white-and-glass IKEA shelves. We also revamped the website and social media accounts and created new messaging.

And people got it. They started to flock in. Okay, they got it for the most part. I did find myself sounding like a robot after ten calls: "Yup, you can just walk in. Nope, you don't need to sign up for a class or book online."

I started working fifteen hours a day, six or seven days a week, and I drove almost forty-five minutes each way to get to the studio. Essentially, I lived at the studio with my puggy and focused one-hundred-percent of my time and effort on the shop. When I wasn't working, I was running around Raleigh picking up paint, toilet paper, wood, glitter, you name it.

I was exhausted but loving every minute. This was what I'd dreamed of when I decided to be my own boss. I was making things happen.

Left foot, right foot, left foot. One morning I was cruising along, crushing miles on the treadmill at the gym, when my phone pinged. An Instagram notification: "Hey, thanks for my gift of stuff from your studio. I'd like to feature you on our news program. Thanks! Annie, ABC News."

Wait, what? I thought. He and I used to watch Annie every morning. *That can't be right. My little studio has only been open a few weeks.*

I'd sent Annie a package filled with goodies from KNACK, including a custom mini wood sign, faux leather earrings, and a bath-bomb cupcake, all packaged in our signature mint color and sent with a handwritten note.

Had it worked? Holy shit.

My heart was racing. *OMG, OMG, OMG. Okay, just stay calm and finish your workout*, I said to myself. *They probably won't stop by for weeks.*

Another ping.

"Are you free at 9:00 a.m. today? We want it for the weekend segment."

OMG OMG OMG. I was a sweaty mess and it was already 8:00 a.m.

"Sure, 9:00 a.m. is perfect."

Not perfect. I need to shower, put on makeup…OMG, I need my good jeans. In the locker room, I called him, so excited that I yelled into the phone, "Get up! Get up! Annie is coming and I can't be on TV without my good jeans. Can you bring them to me NOW?"

Some woman with a stick up her ass asked if I was okay because I was being so loud. I wanted to respond, "Are you okay? Because you're being a jerk! You clearly heard me say I was going to be on the news." Come on, women, let's celebrate each other and not tear each other down.

The jeans in question had been a splurge from Anthropologie at $160 (that's like ten pairs of jeans from Old Navy). They were high waisted with a wide leg and had big pockets in the front and buttons down the sides. They also came with a matching denim belt, and I'd perfected a knotted loop. They looked amazing on me. They looked like, well, $160 jeans. They flowed as I walked and flattered my perfectly flat tummy-tucked stomach.

He had a slight crush on Annie so was happy to drop everything to swing by the shop with my good jeans—otherwise I think I would have been out of luck. He wasn't as keen to be at the shop anymore. And I was starting to notice that I didn't care. But that was for another day.

Lights, camera, action! I was a star!

Okay, maybe that's taking it a little far, but it was a great segment (except for the fact that I was still a little sweaty and had my hair in a slicked-back ponytail). I couldn't believe that the local news was featuring my business within a few weeks of it being open. I hadn't paid a PR firm or a fancy marketing person. It had been all me. I'd trusted my gut and believed in myself.

I thought back to the girl in the meeting worried about her fat rolls, the girl who'd never believed in herself. If I'd told her then that this would be her life in a few short years, she would have laughed and gone back to thinking she was a nobody. A fat nobody.

KNACK quickly became the talk of the town, and I had to hire a team to help keep up, even though the puggy and I were fixtures at the studio.

See, our customers were no longer just people who came to make a project and leave—they had become friends. My entire staff and I knew everyone by name and greeted them warmly as they came through the door. It was like being in an episode of *Cheers*. We celebrated hundreds of birthdays, hosted bridal and baby showers and team-building events. My business philosophy is that people can spend their hard-earned money anywhere, so if they choose to spend it with you, they deserve the best version of you.

The more success the business saw, the more I started doing his duties as well as my own. He seemed to be changing. He listened less and didn't get as excited to celebrate the victories. The more successful the business became, the busier I became, the less I was home, and the less he helped. I was finding my path and building my brand, but we'd started the business together—it was supposed to be *our* thing. Soon he stopped coming by unless I begged for something to be fixed.

At a big VIP kickoff party to celebrate our launch of a new line of projects, he sat in the corner with some staff. He never came to my side. Perhaps I didn't notice because I was so busy. Perhaps he was asking for more and I wasn't there to give it.

The busy times continued. We were doing six to eight birthday parties on Saturdays and Sundays, and the studio was still open for pop-in projects. On Saturdays I'd work from 8:00 a.m. to 11 p.m. without a break (except for a potty break every few hours). I wouldn't eat all day and would then pick up McDonald's on the way home since that's all that was open. I'd also forget to drink water. By the time I got home, all I wanted to do was sleep.

You hear it all the time: to get the glory, you need to put in the work. The work was paying off—my news segment ran eight times over two days (even I got sick of seeing my face, but I was very grateful); I was in a book about women leaders in Raleigh; I sat on several panels; I was a keynote speaker; I had a dedicated, awesome team of ten; the studio was turning a profit within the first few months—everything was great. But I have this horrible habit of focusing on one goal and letting everything else fall by the wayside. People have often looked at me and said, "Wow, she's doing so great." Meanwhile, the rest of my life is falling apart around me.

I was packing on the pounds from my crappy eating, late nights, and, oh, did I mention that all the people who held birthday parties at the studio generously offered us cake? There were weekends I was eating three to five pieces of delicious, creamy, mouthwatering cake a day. I have now tried something from every bakery with a ten-mile radius of the studio. If you're in Raleigh and need a cake suggestion, I'm your girl.

My pants got a little tighter. And tighter. And…shit. Fuck. *My stupid paint jeans don't even fit anymore. Yup, they just ripped on the inner thigh. Am I going to wear yoga pants to work now?*

I had no energy the moment I left the studio, and my relationship was crumbling. He needed more of me and I couldn't give it. So, after a year and a half, I decided that even though I loved what I did, I'd list the business for sale.

This was a novel idea at the time—who would want to buy a brand-new business with only one-and-a-half years' proof of concept? But we were doing all the right things: we had a strong online presence, experienced staff, and good community presence. In a world of dying retail, we offered an experience, something that couldn't be bought online.

It was a tough decision, but I'd become someone I didn't recognize, and not just because of the weight. I was starting to slip back into the depths of sadness. I was fighting with him all the time, until he didn't even care to fight anymore. I needed to regain my strength. I needed to rediscover me.

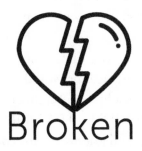

Broken

"I'm dead inside. I don't love you, or anyone. I just need to be alone."

His words cut through me like a dagger. I had no response. My heart sank into my stomach. I felt sick. I blacked out for a moment and everything slowed down, just as it had when I was handed the seat-belt extender. I'd known we were struggling but had hoped a new day would bring new life to our new love.

The passion had died. The affection was gone. It had taken me over thirty-five years to find love, and in the blink of an eye, it was ending.

I had no idea what to do, where to go. I'd moved in a year ago. With my eyes almost swollen shut from crying, I grabbed my puggy and my purse, got into the car, and started driving aimlessly.

And then I called my mom.

Pick up, pick up…

"Hello?"

"He…l…oh," *sniffle*. Bursting into tears.

"Dina, what happened? Where are you? Take a breath."

Hyperventilating.

"It's over." That sentence would take me several minutes to get out.

"What happened…?"

"He's dead inside and doesn't love me anymore…"

This man I'd loved so much, this man I'd wanted to spend the rest of my life with, who'd taken care of me during my surgery, who'd changed my bandages, who'd made me grilled cheese sandwiches naked, who'd cuddled me, who'd shared a home with me, who'd said I was the most beautiful woman and the best thing that had happened to him DIDN'T LOVE ME ANYMORE.

What had happened? I'd lost myself, my confidence, my fearlessness, my independence, my strength. Right from the beginning, I craved him like a drug. Before I started KNACK, I'd sit at my corporate job and lose focus because I was thinking about him. He'd become my addiction, so much so that I turned a blind eye to his bad behavior.

All I could think about in that moment were the good times. I forgot about the bad times. About the way he turned everything into my fault. I forgot about how I apologized for things I shouldn't have been sorry for, like using cooking spray instead of butter when making eggs. About how lately, he only seemed to love me when he was drinking. About how he lied about and tried to hide his drinking but made me feel like an asshole for asking about it. About how he barely wanted to talk to me anymore. About how he stopped sharing anything about his world, and how when I asked about it, he'd get annoyed.

I somehow found myself at the Starbucks drive-through. I couldn't remember driving there. The sweet girl in the window looked at my red, puffy, ugly-crying eyes, the tears streaming down my face, and my puggy in the passenger seat looking at me with so much love and confusion, and then said the kindest words to me: "I'm not sure what you're going through, but just know everything will be okay. I'm sure you're a good person and you'll come through this. Your coffee is on me." Sometimes I think about my Starbucks angel and wonder if that really happened or I just dreamed it.

It was just a few weeks before our two-year anniversary. Only two years, but I had made him my world—maybe too much so. Like Selena Gomez says in her song "Lose You to Love Me," I let him come first and he loved it.

The next morning, I woke to find the sun shining down on me as I lay on my couch in the loft, where we kept all the stuff from my apartment, my former life. It were as though he'd created a living storage unit for me until he was done with me, as though I were a placeholder until that someone he cared for from his past finally chose him.

It was the red flag I'd been ignoring.

I hadn't trusted her from the beginning, but he'd assured me it was my imagination, just me being "insecure and crazy."

It was a beautiful day outside but all I wanted to do was sleep and cry. My head was pounding from crying all night. Not even *Friends* had been able to bring a smile to my face. He never came to check on me

I bet he's sleeping like a baby.

I headed to the master bedroom, gently opened the door so it wouldn't creak, and tip-toed to the foot of the bed. He looked peaceful and comfortable in our king-sized bed, his foot peeking out from under the white comforter that I'd paid for, as if a weight had been lifted off his shoulders.

He'd gotten rid of me and now had the freedom to love her. In that moment, I knew he was done and there was no turning back for him.

I promised myself that I wouldn't let this relationship continue to define me. He'd made me feel stupid, as if everything that had happened were a story I'd created in my head. I'd started to doubt myself—hell, I'd flat-out blamed myself for everything wrong with our relationship. And all along, I'd been dating a master manipulator.

I've said it before: rage and determination will get you far in life. It doesn't mean I don't feel the hurt—it just means that when I have a broken heart, I'm able to put on my big-girl pants and save the crying for another day.

The next day, after a long day at work, I walked through the door and said to him, "I found an apartment, and I'll be out in a week." He'd clearly underestimated me and forgotten the strong, independent women he'd fallen in love with, as he seemed shocked and stumbled over his words. "Well, you don't have to leave so quick. You can stay here for a little bit, save up, blah blah blah…"

Nope, I'm good, thanks. All I could think was *I'd rather sleep in my car.*

That was the last time I'd ever see him.

Everything I'd worked for had come crashing down: my health, my relationship, my passion for my business (it was supposed to have been ours, remember). My world was in a million pieces. All I could do was tell myself over and over that life in this moment was temporary.

I resolved that I would find another place for me and the puggy to call home longer term, to continue to list the business for sale, to find a new job that I could get excited about, and, well…to find and love myself again.

Meantime, I cried and unpacked at the new apartment I'd found so quickly and leaned on friends and laughed and cried and ate tacos and listened to Eddie and his sad songs and cried and cried.

One day, after crying for about an hour, I saw this quote online:

"She remembered who she was and the game changed," Lalah Delia.

And just like that, the pity party for one was over. I put on my running shoes. This would be my therapy.

My shoes were dusty. The only action they'd seen lately was the inside of a moving box. The soles were worn, but from races I'd run long ago. The last time I'd put on these shoes, almost a year earlier, I was pulled off the half-marathon course in Virginia Beach by the slagging wagon. It was the first time I'd ever been pulled. I hadn't been ready mentally, emotionally, or physically that day.

As I walked down each step of my new apartment, I told myself, "Today is day one. You're a new you, the best you, the strongest you. You're a fighter."

I had no idea where I was going or how long I'd be gone—I just wanted to clear my head. I'd been running for years on and off and had never really loved it. I loved the idea of it but not the work it took.

This time, it was different. It wasn't about how fast my mile was, or how far I ran. This time, it was about healing my heart and finding myself. As I ran, I processed things.

I started running every day. I couldn't wait to hit the open road, just me and my thoughts. I got stronger and faster, and as the tears dried up, I recognized that my thoughts had been shifting from lost love to rebuilding and rediscovering myself.

I created a playlist of all the songs that built me up, including "The Fighter," by Keith Urban and Carrie Underwood, "Can't Hold Us," by Macklemore and Ryan Lewis, and "Sorry" by the Queen Bee (Beyoncé) herself.

I ran my heart out, mile after mile, and when Lizzo's "Good as Hell"—my anthem, my mantra, my favorite song—came on, I shouted the words from the top of my lungs.

Because in that moment on the greenway, with the sun beating down on me, sweat dripping down my face and my shirt soaked as though I'd just gotten out of the shower, I realized, "I do deserve to feel good as hell!"

Part Three:
Your Journey to
I Am

"What if I fall?"
"Oh but my darling, what if you fly?"
Erin Hanson

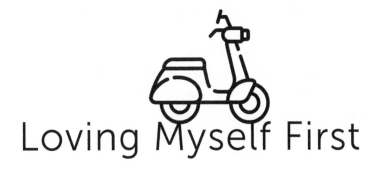

Loving Myself First

Rebuilding and rediscovering yourself means walking a long, hard road. You need to be committed and you also need to give yourself grace. I struggled so much trying to understand this simple idea. If I'd heard someone speak to someone else the way I used to speak to myself, I would have been offended, but yet, I was doing it.

I knew that rebuilding wouldn't be easy or fast. I knew it needed to become a lifestyle. I'm a visual person, so I wanted an image that I could think of that would remind me to stay focused.

I chose the image of a Vespa.

It's made for one person, gets you to where you need to go but not fast, and doesn't have a lot of room for baggage.

I wanted to set goals and track them but also didn't want to start with too many and end up shutting down. I researched tons of motivating practices but couldn't find one that fit.

So, I started by simply breaking down my life into the five areas that caused me the most stress but could result in the most happiness if done right: career, love, health and fitness, self + care, and finances.

At first, the list felt overwhelming. *How the hell am I going to put my life back together given how many of these things have fallen apart?* I knew I couldn't tackle it all at once.

My heart was broken into a million pieces, so I took love off the table. That was a start.

I had found myself a steady, good-paying job that was perfect for the moment, and I still kept up with the business for a few months. I needed to be in a role where I could get shit done but also be somewhat checked out, a role where no one was checking in on me, so I found a job in which my manager was three thousand miles away! Check...for now.

My finances were a disaster, as I'd not received a check for a year—one of the struggles of business ownership. Sorting this area out was a must, no matter how much I didn't want to do it!

My archenemy FAT was back, and seemingly with a vengeance—I thought I looked like shit, and I felt even shittier. The crappy food I'd been eating during my KNACK days had not only made me fat but had also made my skin dull and lifeless and my hair lose its shine. I was a mess. Health and fitness also needed to be on the list.

The last to make the list was self + care—the easiest one, right? I figured I'd get a few facials and manis and pedis and have a few girls' nights. Check, check.

Boy, did I get a big-ass punch in the face when I realized what self + care actually was (which I'll get to shortly).

Once I knew what I needed (or thought I needed) to do, I needed to figure out how to do it. I had to create a time frame, a deadline.

Hmmm, well, thirty days is too short to build anything more than a foundation, and a year is too long to stay motivated. I mean, I fell totally in and out of love in two years, so...

I decided that I'd break my life into ninety-day segments. *Yeah, ninety days.* During each segment, I committed to tackling a different area.

And so, I hopped on my imaginary Vespa with three bags for the next ninety days: health and fitness, finances, and self + care. I knew this was a lot to tackle, so I started slow. I would create a foundation and build from there. I reminded myself, *This is my journey. It's all about me.* Someone I forgot about a while ago.

I created a list of basics to get me started and shared my journey on Instagram as a way to hold myself accountable.

Things to Tackle:

- Run three times a week
- Get a budget together
- Do one nice, self + care thing for myself every week

Okay, I was kind of cheating with running, since I'd started running a few weeks earlier, so I added a little extra to this goal right away: I signed up for a 5k that was two months away. My goal was to beat my fastest finish-time to date (fifty-five minutes) and complete it in fifty minutes. I know, I know, runners, I hear you—this is not fast for six-minute milers, but remember, my Vespa, my goals, so get out of my way!

Feeling focused and good—good as hell, actually, I decided to push it further. I would put aside my insecurities about my running speed and not being good enough and would find a running group.

Race entry paid for Labor Day, exactly one year after my failed half marathon…check. Running group found…check.

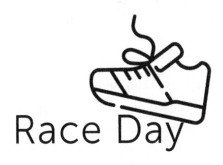

Race Day

I confidently laced up my new Cinderella-blue New Balance sneakers, fired up my running playlist, set my watch, and waited for the gun.

I started out strong, confident, found someone to keep pace with, finished my first mile one minute under my goal mile time, hit the turnaround point, and saw a slew of people behind me. More times than not in my running history, I'd been near the end. And during my first 10k, several years earlier, I was dead last. That day, the people on the pace bikes in front of me kept telling me I needed to keep my pace or I'd be pulled, and a police officer on a motorcycle behind me cheered me on. His face was covered in a ski mask to protect him from the cold, so only his gentle dark brown eyes showed. "Come on," he said encouragingly. "You can do this. We're almost there." In that moment, I had two choices: give in to my embarrassment and give up or find my strength and finish strong. *Fuck it*, I thought. *I have nothing to lose now.* I had to get back to the finish line anyway, since my car was there. So I turned to the officer, gestured to the cavalcade around me, and said, "Is this what the president feels like when he's running?" I finished last to the sound of the crowd's cheering—cheering because I'd done it. I'd done it.

The Labor Day race was an improvement, to say the least. In

fact, I crushed my goal by two minutes. I couldn't believe it. I'd set a goal, worked my ass off, and it had paid off. I was on top of the moon.

Just a few weeks after my race, I walked into the store where I'd bought my new running shoes. This time, I was nervous and intimidated, not excited. It was the first day with my new running group, with whom I'd spend every Thursday and Saturday for the next ten weeks. The moment I met the coaches and mentors, I knew I'd made the right decision. There were two coaches, and both were warm and welcoming. One was funny and spunky—and a little silly, like me—and the other was calm and collected. She made sure to capture every moment of the journey, and they both cheered on and encouraged each runner with every ounce of energy they had.

The mentors had so many tips and tricks. Whenever I run now, I have the words of one of them in my head: stand up straight, hold your box, and don't crush the baby chicks. I repeated this over and over as I ran. Soon, I couldn't wait for Thursdays and Saturdays, when I'd get to see my teammates, my friends.

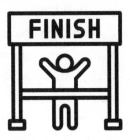

Target: Chicago

I decided to set a bigger goal: I was going to run the Chicago Marathon, which was taking place exactly nine days after my thirty-ninth birthday. I had a year to train—plenty of time. Because running a marathon seemed like an impossible dream, I decided to make running a main focus for the next six segments in my ninety-day plan, maybe more. Running had become such a big part of my life I couldn't imagine not doing it at this point.

During this time, Amazon Studios released a movie that could have been about my life. *Brittany Runs a Marathon* spoke to every fiber of my being. If you haven't seen it, watch it. If you're not a runner, apply the message to anything you've thought you could never do.

I was focusing on other goals during my ninety-day segments at this time as well, notably finances. In ninety days, I'd listed and sold KNACK in what I consider record time—eighteen days after I'd listed it—I landed a new gig at a startup and I was living on my own again (in a swanky apartment).

I've always been the breadwinner; I feel comfortable with it. I made double my ex-husband and carried the burden of that for years. And years later, I leaned on someone for the first time ever—I leaned on "him" when I opened the studio. I think he liked it. With his ex-wife, he'd been the one bringing home the bacon, and he'd struggled a little knowing how much I made.

It seems crazy to me that in this day and age, some men still can't handle making less than a woman. I used to joke that men say they want a strong, independent woman until they meet one in real life. Then they run for the hills!

I hated the feeling of being taken care of. He used it as a form of control. I had to ask to spend money and felt guilty if I did. I stopped shopping, getting my hair cut (I went nine months without a haircut), buying less expensive makeup, etcetera.

But now it was all back on me: rent, car, phone, puggy meds, Internet, gas, food, and on and on. I needed to get on track. I had things I needed to save for, adventures I wanted to take. I'd planned an action-packed year and wanted to figure out a way to meet my goals without racking up debt.

For the first time, I had a budget and I was sticking to it.

I'd stumbled upon a woman on Instagram, The Budget Mom, who used the cash-envelope system. I downloaded her envelopes, read her blog, which details her financial struggles and how she's gotten to where she is today, and decided to take my finances by the balls and make them my bitch. I created envelopes for gas, groceries, puggy, hair, nails, me, miscellaneous, car maintenance, and girls' nights out. I started paying all my bills online. I made a list of expenses and when they were due—cell phone, water, rent, Netflix, Hulu, gym, etc.—and a list of debt payments and when they were due—credit cards, car payment, etc. Seeing how expensive my life had become was a real eye-opener.

I created a plan to clear the debt and started using only cash wherever I could. The way some people looked at me when I paid for things in cash, you'd think I was writing out a check. I could almost hear people behind me in line at the grocery store huffing under their breath. I wanted to say, "Listen here, asshole, I'm on a damn budget, so back off."

My other financial goals were to start a savings account and build a new wardrobe as I rebuilt my body and transitioned back into the corporate world. I wanted financial freedom and to live debt free. It would take two ninety-day cycles to get my footing, and then budgeting became an automatic process for me. With everything in place, it became a simple copy and paste every month.

Self + care was by far the hardest area of focus for me. It could have been a sole focus for several blocks of ninety days. As mentioned, I'd thought it would be the easiest—just go get pampered and take time for myself. But I would quickly see it wasn't self-care but self + care. And truly, self + love. I would learn how to care for myself.

I devoured all things female empowerment, including my idol Rachel Hollis's books, *Girl, Wash Your Face* (twice) and *Girl, Stop Apologizing*. I also watched her daily live video.

The big question in my mind was, *How do I find peace?*

Reflecting on the thirty-eight years of my life, and especially the last eight, I came to realize that not only did I not have self + love, I actually had lots and lots of self + hate. Self + hate had led me to a loveless marriage, to binge-eating, to falling in love with a narcissist, to destroying friendships, to destroying me. I'd let people I truly cared for slip out of my life because of stupid things, such as my feeling unaccepted by them. Over the years I'd had many, many moments of happiness and laughter. I'd had a great life, but the truth was I'd let my self + hate define so many moments.

The more I ran, the more peace I found. I learned I didn't need to be on the go all the time. I wanted to sit, reflect, read (I read more books in that time than in all the years of my life combined), watch Netflix, work on my word-search puzzles (yup, prepping for my senior years), and eat cereal for dinner if I wanted (I know, it went against the health goal, but sometimes you need a splurge). I learned how to be alone with my thoughts.

I learned how to be alone.

I found happiness in solitude for the first time. Of course, my therapist received many visits. I became "selfish" and put me first. OMG yes, this people pleaser, never-say-no enthusiast, over-achiever PUT HERSELF FIRST! I realized I was a better friend, daughter, employee, hell, even a better stranger on the street when my needs were met. Saying no to things was super hard, but I just kept picturing myself on the Vespa.

Once I had the ninety-day timeframe, I wondered how I'd ever jump the hurdles in front of me. The key was to take the process day by day. There were no do-overs, no restarts—just the ninety days and me.

I told myself it was okay to have missteps. I wouldn't consider them mistakes, just speed bumps in the journey. I told myself, *Life isn't perfect, and I'm not perfect. My imperfections make me who I am.*

I'd started sharing my journey on Instagram just for me, to hold myself accountable, but I couldn't believe the encouragement I received—so many positive messages from women just like me. Women who were struggling on their own journeys and wanted to do their own ninety days. They turned to me for advice. Me. The person who just years before had been so sad, had cried over a seat-belt extender, had lived a loveless life. Me.

Before I knew it, I was eighty days in and needed to start thinking about the goals for the next ninety days. And my first ninety days finished right around my birthday, so it was a double celebration.

I had a "day of me." I got a new haircut and style (which might be my best hairstyle ever). And a new pair of jeans—a new brand at Target: dark-wash, dressy jeans with a wide leg and high waist. I also found the most amazing blush in pink (my favorite color) and a pleather motorcycle jacket that was cut for my curves. That night, I celebrated in style with my girlfriends at a local spot where we could sit outside and bask in the gorgeous October night. We laughed and enjoyed great food and yummy drinks, just like Reese and Sandra and Scarlett.

I'd always felt that I had a calling to lift, motivate, and inspire others. I'd always felt I was put here with a higher purpose. But over the years I'd wondered, *How can I be that person when my own journey isn't even close to perfect? Hell, it's downright messy!*

What I've learned through this journey, though, is that throughout the mess, there have been moments of all kinds: moments of joy, sadness, love, and loss. And because I've gone through them all, I'm able to motivate those around me. My imperfection is real, honest, and sometimes hard to hear about. It's what drives me to do better. It's the foundation of what built me.

Your *I Am* Journey

Welcome to your *I Am* journey! It's time to take back control of your life, ninety days at a time. Hop on your Vespa and start your *I Am* journey. This journey is all about you. It's all about discovering who you are and living your best life.

Let's get this straight: I'm not a doctor or a nutritionist or a therapist or a personal trainer. What I am is a woman who's been on a journey of self-discovery for the last twenty years. I've read hundreds of books and magazine articles, attended numerous lectures and seminars, and could probably teach some of the authors and speakers a thing or two. What all the advice boils down to is one fundamental principle: *If you don't love yourself, you can't love anyone or anything else properly.*

What is *I Am*? *I Am* is your new mantra. *I Am* will guide your journey. With every goal you set, ask yourself "Is this an *I Am* goal?" Ask yourself, "Is my goal **I**mpactful, **A**chievable, and **M**eaningful?"

Impactful: It has a major effect

Think of your goal as a force. YOU ARE A FORCE! Many of us tend to say yes to everything and spread ourselves too thin, which leads us to give up on our goals. Learn to say NO. Focus on saying yes only to things that will have a big positive impact on your life. What effects are your goals having on your life? If your goal is in health and fitness, what does a new healthy diet and/or exercise routine mean for you? What impact do you want it to have on your life? Do you want to lose weight or lower your cholesterol or wean yourself off a particular medication? Or do you want to feel mentally alert, stronger, and more in control of your body? Do you want to live longer? Consider the impact.

Achievable: It can be brought about

Setting goals that are achievable can be the most difficult part of the process. It's easy to come up with a goal and then hit the ground running full speed out of the gate only to lose stamina in thirty days or less. I like to call this "goal burnout." Remember, you have the ability to expand on a goal twelve times during the ninety days. So, if you're currently not exercising at all, for example, don't make it your goal to run three miles at an eight-minute-per-mile pace in your first week. You might start with walk-run intervals for a set time. Keep building gradually each week while continuing to push so as not to get stale.

Meaningful: It's important to you and adds value to your life in some way

Living your life with purpose means making sure you're creating meaningful moments. These are the moments that matter. These are the moments we slow down to stop and appreciate.

When setting a goal, consider why it matters. Is your career where you want to create the most meaning right now, so you can provide a better life for your family? Or do you want to focus on your finances so you can be debt free or buy a house or take a dream vacation? There's no point in creating goals if they don't mean anything. Where will you be ninety days from now if you don't start today? What about a year from now?

This journey will challenge you to dig deep to find what matters most to you, especially in the moments of stress, weakness, and doubt. These are your moments to shine, to rise up and take control of your goals and your life.

Remember it's ninety days, for good or bad. We don't get to erase days in real life, so you don't get to erase them here. Here's how it works.

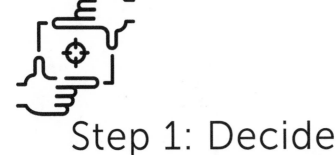

Step 1: Decide

Decide where you'll direct your focus: finances, love, health and fitness, self + care, or career. Choose no more than three areas, so you don't get overwhelmed (and feel free to choose only one). There may be some areas of your life that require just a little fine-tuning. Other areas might be a total shit show. You do you! You know better than anyone what you can handle and where you can push.

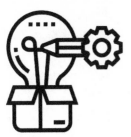

Step 2: Create

Create a weekly goal and plan of action for ninety days. You'll find a link where you can download your own goal-setting worksheets at the end of this book, but here's what they look like.

Dina Marie

Goal Setting
AREA OF FOCUS: HEALTH + FITNESS

END GOAL - 90 DAYS

Week 1 Goal + Plan of Action

Week 2 Goal + Plan of Action

Week 3 Goal + Plan of Action

Week 4 Goal + Plan of Action

i am

Week 5 Goal + Plan of Action

Week 6 Goal + Plan of Action

Week 7 Goal + Plan of Action

Week 8 Goal + Plan of Action

Week 9 Goal + Plan of Action

i am

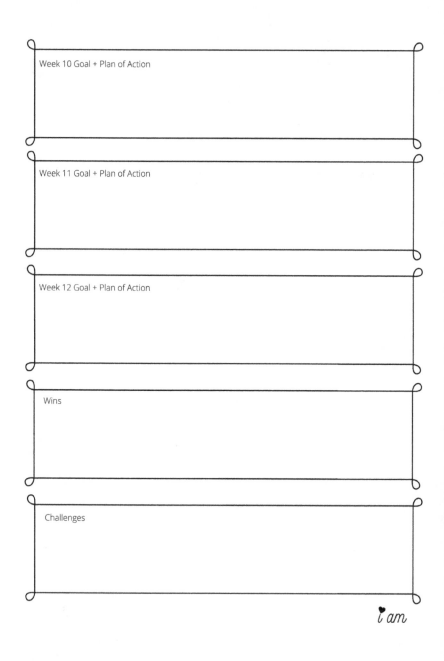

Week 10 Goal + Plan of Action

Week 11 Goal + Plan of Action

Week 12 Goal + Plan of Action

Wins

Challenges

i am

Don't work on the details of a weekly goal more than two weeks ahead of time. It's okay to have a general outline of goals you want to hit each week, but avoid building in details too far in advance because if you fall behind or get ahead, you might end up adding unnecessary obstacles to your journey.

Find fifteen minutes a week for planning. Mark it on your calendar or set an alarm on your phone—whatever it takes to find at least fifteen minutes a week to work on your goals and plan of action. I know, I know, you have so much going on in your life, and finding fifteen minutes could be tricky, but if you have decided "I am worth it," you'll find the time.

Feel free to create an end goal and build your weekly plan accordingly, working backward. And get creative with your goals! They can be incorporated over as many cycles as you want—you don't have to finish them in ninety days. For example, I'm training for a marathon, so my running goals (under health and fitness) will be present for six cycles of ninety days. I create a plan for each ninety-day segment. I also try not to copy and paste the goal into each cycle, as I want to get better and faster. After I finish the marathon, running will still be part of my life but may not be a goal that requires a detailed plan.

Here's a look at what a sample ninety-day plan looks like when it's completed.

Goal Setting

AREA OF FOCUS: HEALTH + FITNESS

SAMPLE

END GOAL - 90 DAYS

Complete a 5K by the end of the 90 days
Goal Race: Pretend Race Name

Week 1 Goal + Plan of Action

Find a local 5K Race
Get fitted for New shoes
Walk for 30 minutes for 3 days

Week 2 Goal + Plan of Action

Download couch to 5K app
Follow app's Recommended activity, 3 days a week 15-
25 minutes walk/Run intervals

Week 3 Goal + Plan of Action

Try a New trail to walk/Run
Find a buddy to train with
App 3 days- 25-30 minutes walk/Run intervals

Week 4 Goal + Plan of Action

Add weights 1 day per week
Find weight training workouts on pinterest
App 3 days- 25-30 minutes walk/Run intervals

i am

Week 5 Goal + Plan of Action
Add weights 2 days per week
Reduce sugar from diet
App 3 days— 25-30 minutes walk/run intervals

Week 6 Goal + Plan of Action
Add 2 new vegetables to diet
Sign up for race
App 3 days— 25-30 minutes walk/run intervals

Week 7 Goal + Plan of Action
Find a new training buddy since yours flaked out
Continue weights 2 days per week
App 3 days— 25-30 minutes walk/run intervals

Week 8 Goal + Plan of Action
Get a new sports bra and running pants
weights 1 day/week + add swimming 1 day/week
App 3 days— 30-35 minutes walk/run longer intervals

Week 9 Goal + Plan of Action
Set a race day goal time
find a cheering squad for your 1st race
App 3 days— 30-35 minutes walk/run longerintervals

i am

Week 10 Goal + Plan of Action

Try New Running hydration— Noom, etc
App 3 days— 35-40 minutes walk/run longer intervals

Week 11 Goal + Plan of Action

Test pre-run dinner
Begin to taper based on app

Week 12 Goal + Plan of Action

Get a good night sleep
RACE DAY!!!! Celebrate!!!!

Wins

Completed 5 k in under my goal time!
Lost 5 lbs in the process
Added 2 or more vegetables to every meal

Challenges

Still consuming sugar
Did not relax properly on rest days

i am

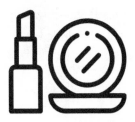

Step 3: Write

Now it's time to write your *I Am* mantra. Write it in a journal, put it on the bathroom mirror with lipstick, type it up and frame it—I don't care, just do something with it!

Look in the mirror and say it out loud every day for at least thirty days. Say it with conviction, say it loud and proud, hell, shout the damn words! These words will become your strength when you feel like giving up—when you don't feel like exercising or when you feel like soothing yourself with sugar after a bad day or blowing your savings on a Louis Vuitton handbag. In the moments when you're faced with a fork in the road, SHOUT your mantra over and over until you remember to trust and believe in yourself.

Find a mantra that's all yours, and don't change it until it becomes a habit or a part of you. Here are a few examples:

I AM STRONG
I AM POWERFUL
I AM ENOUGH
I AM BEAUTIFUL
I AM SMART
I AM SUCCESSFUL
I AM A FORCE
I AM UNSTOPPABLE

Head on over to justmedinamarie.com/collections/digital-downloads to download your very own set of the worksheets I've included in this book to keep yourself on track!

The Pants That No Longer Define Me

Today, in a neat three-crease fold, in the closet, are the pants that, in 2011, I thought defined me as a person on the saddest day of my life.

Today, I look at these pants with a sense of pride and accomplishment. I went on a journey of love and heartbreak, and at the end of the road, I achieved something I'd always struggled with: I learned to love myself first.

And so finally, we come to love. I'd told myself I wouldn't think about love in my first several ninety-day segments. I wanted to find peace with being alone, both in my head and in my heart. And I did.

Now, in this new decade, on Valentine's Day, as I sit in a café in Berlin, Germany, with tea and a pretzel (man, the Germans love their carbs), I look out into the sea of people and realize that my heart will be ready for love again—soon.

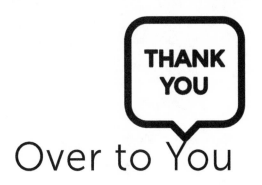

Over to You

If you enjoyed *My Fat Pants Don't Fit*, please consider leaving a brief review on the website or with the retailer where you bought the book.

Reviews are very important to every author. Your feedback doesn't have to be long or detailed. Just a sentence saying what you enjoyed.

Please accept my thanks in advance.

Acknowledgements

Writing a book seemed like a daunting task for me, someone who hates to write even an email. But as the words flowed out, I started thinking about all the people who supported, loved, and carried me through my journey to self + love and this book.

None of this would have been possible without the team at Ingenium Books: my editor Rachel Small, who turned my words into a real story, and publisher Boni Wagner-Stafford, who spent hours with me on video chat making sure my voice would be heard.

To my mom, Diane Shaffer, who is my rock, my best friend, my biggest cheerleader, and an all-around badass. Through tears and laughter she has been by my side, inspiring me to become the woman I am today.

To Dan Clossey, my mentor, friend, and sounding board. You have always believed in me and my crazy dreams. You encouraged and pushed me to be the strongest version of myself.

To JV, who spent thousands of hours of listening and guiding but never judging. I am thankful for you and would not be this version of me without you.

To all the women in my life that have listened to my stories, shared in my moments, gave advice, and loved me for me! You have been in the thick of this journey and you stuck by my side. You get me!

About the Author

Dina Marie is a two time, badass #girlboss entrepreneur, creating Delish Gourmet Bath Bakery and KNACK DIY Craft Studio. In the corporate world she has dominated recruiting efforts for small to mid-size startups.

She is a motivational keynote speaker with a fun, energetic, raw, and infectious delivery of stories about life after divorce, extreme weight loss, falling in love—only to have her heart broken into a million pieces—before ultimately finding self-love. Dina continues to build and support the community of amazing women that want to take the leap to create the life of their dreams.

Dina is a proud dog mom to her precious pug, Bean. She is a city girl at heart, calling downtown Durham, North Carolina her home.

CPSIA information can be obtained
at www.ICGtesting.com
Printed in the USA
LVHW111610040620
657378LV00005B/294